Weight Watch New Complete Cookbook 2024

Simple, Healthy & Delicious Recipes to Support Your Weight Loss Goals and Enhance Your Healthy Living

By

Dr. Eva R. Alonzo

TABLE OF CONTENT

CONCLUSION 93

Greetings and welcome to the "Weight Watch New Complete Cookbook 2024," a cooking manual created to motivate, encourage, and enable you on your path to a healthier way of life. This cookbook is more than just a list of recipes; it's an endorsement of the idea that eating healthfully can be fulfilling and life-changing.

A dedication to well-being

At Weight Watchers, we recognize that reaching and keeping a healthy weight requires making sustainable, wise decisions over the course of a lifetime. This cookbook has been painstakingly designed to be consistent with the principles of the Weight Watchers program, which prioritize variety, balance, and enjoying food. Every dish is meant to provide you with tasty, fulfilling meals and support you in achieving your objectives.

Investigating Diversity in Culinary Arts

The variety of cuisines included in this cookbook is one of its best qualities. We've collected recipes from all around the world to infuse your kitchen with a diverse range of tastes and culinary traditions. There is something for every palate, from the bright, fresh foods of the Mediterranean to the cozy, filling dinners influenced by classic American cooking. These recipes are straightforward and versatile, so it doesn't matter if you are an experienced chef or a kitchen novice—making delicious dinners for your family is simple.

Stressing Taste and Nutrition

Flavor should never have to be sacrificed in the name of health. We take great effort in creating our recipes to make sure that each bite is both delicious and nourishing. Whole, fresh ingredients that are bursting with flavor and minerals are our top priority. We may make meals that are higher in satisfaction but lower in calories by concentrating on these elements. Maintaining your health goals is made easier with the inclusion of Weight Watcher point values and comprehensive nutritional information in every recipe.

Assisting you on your journey

The purpose of this cookbook is to assist you in your efforts to improve your health and lose weight. We are aware that creating long-lasting changes can be difficult, but having a selection of delectable, simple recipes at your disposal can help a lot. "Weight Watch New Complete Cookbook 2024" provides a variety of dishes for all occasions, including big dinners and decadent desserts, as well as quick breakfasts and light lunches. You can stick to your health objectives and yet enjoy your favorite foods with these recipes.

Creating Long-Term Routines

Our strategy is based on the idea that creating enduring eating habits—rather than imposing restrictions or deprivation—is the key to good eating. This cookbook's recipes are designed to foster a healthy relationship between you and food, allowing you to enjoy preparing and eating meals without feeling guilty or under pressure. We offer cooking, purchasing, and meal planning advice that will make it easy for you to include these dishes into your regular routine.

A Well-Being Community

Selecting this cookbook also means that you're a part of a community that celebrates wellness, health, and the joy of delicious cuisine. Since community support is the cornerstone of the Weight Watch program, we want you to tell others about your cooking adventures, triumphs, and even setbacks. As a team, we can encourage and inspire one another to keep moving forward and accomplish our objectives.

Gazing Forward

This "Weight Watch New Complete Cookbook 2024" is simply the start of an exciting trip filled with tasty food. We hope that as you try these recipes, you'll discover new favorites that you'll keep on hand in your kitchen. Take this cookbook as a guide to try new recipes, play around with different ingredients, and most of all, have fun preparing and eating a balanced meal.

Last Words

We appreciate you selecting the "Weight Watch New Complete Cookbook 2024" to be your cooking partner. We can't wait to help you on your journey to a better, happier version of yourself by sharing these recipes with you. Cheers to a year full of flavorful dishes, satisfying cooking, and the satisfaction that comes with eating and cooking well.

------ RECIPES ------

BLUEBERRY BANANA PANCAKES

Prep Time: 10 min

Cook Time: 15 min

Servings: 4 (2 pancakes per serving)

Points Values: 4 per serving

Ingredients:

- 1 cup of whole wheat flour
- 1 tsp baking powder
- 1/2 tsp baking soda
- 1/4 tsp salt
- 1 cup of unsweetened almond milk
- 1 large egg
- 1 medium ripe banana, mashed
- 1/2 cup of fresh blueberries
- Cooking spray

Instructions:

1. Mix the flour, baking soda, baking powder, and salt in a big bowl.
2. Blend almond milk, egg, and mashed banana until smooth in another bowl.
3. Mix the dry ingredients with the wet ones until they are barely mixed.
4. Fold in blueberries gently.
5. Apply cooking spray to a nonstick skillet and heat it over medium heat.
6. For every pancake, add 1/4 cup of batter to the skillet. Cook until surface bubbles appear, then turn and continue cooking until golden brown.
7. Warm up and serve.

Nutrition Info (per serving):

Calories: 150

Protein: 6g Carbs: 28g Fat: 3g Fiber: 4g

Prep Time: 10 min

Cook Time: 10 min

Servings: 1

Points Values: 3 per serving

Ingredients:

- 2 large eggs
- 1/4 cup of chop-up bell peppers
- 1/4 cup of chop-up tomatoes
- 1/4 cup of chop-up spinach
- 1/4 cup of split mushrooms
- 1/4 cup of diced onions
- Cooking spray
- Salt and pepper to taste

Instructions:

1. In a bowl, whisk together eggs and add pepper and salt to taste.
2. Apply cooking spray to a nonstick skillet and heat it over medium heat.
3. Sauté onions, bell peppers, tomatoes, spinach, and mushrooms until they become tender.
4. Over the veggies in the skillet, pour the eggs.
5. Fold the omelet in half after cooking until the eggs are set.
6. Serve right away.

Nutrition Info (per serving):

Calories: 180

Protein: 14g

Carbs: 6g

Fat: 12g

Fiber: 2g

Prep Time: 5 min

Cook Time: 0 min

Servings: 1

Points Values: 4 per serving

Ingredients:

- 1 cup of non-fat Greek yogurt
- 1/2 cup of mixed fresh berries
- 1 tbsp honey
- 2 tbsp granola

Instructions:

1. Arrange half of the yogurt into a glass or bowl.
2. Pour in half of the honey and half of the mixed berries.
3. With the leftover yogurt, berries, and honey, repeat the layering process.
4. Sprinkle granola on top.
5. Serve right away.

Nutrition Info (per serving):

Calories: 220

Protein: 14g

Carbs: 35g

Fat: 2g

Fiber: 5g

Prep Time: 5 min

Cook Time: 5 min

Servings: 1

Points Values: 5 per serving

Ingredients:

- 1 whole wheat tortilla
- 1/2 cup of fresh spinach
- 1/4 cup of crumbled feta cheese
- 2 large eggs
- Cooking spray

Instructions:

1. Apply cooking spray to a nonstick skillet and heat it over medium heat.
2. Cook the spinach in the skillet until it wilts.
3. Pour the whisked eggs into a basin over the skillet of spinach. Cook the eggs until they are thoroughly cooked and scrambled, stirring from time to time.
4. Arrange the spinach and scrambled eggs in the middle of the tortilla, top with feta cheese, and then fold it up.
5. Serve right away.

Nutrition Info (per serving):

Calories: 250

Protein: 18g

Carbs: 20g

Fat: 10g

Fiber: 3g

Prep Time: 10 min

Cook Time: 0 min (overnight refrigeration)

Servings: 1

Points Values: 5 per serving

Ingredients:

- 1/2 cup of rolled oats
- 1/2 cup of unsweetened almond milk
- 1/4 cup of unsweetened applesauce
- 1/4 cup of diced apple
- 1/2 tsp ground cinnamon
- 1 tsp chia seeds (non-compulsory)
- 1 tsp honey

Instructions:

1. Oats, almond milk, applesauce, split apple, cinnamon, and chia seeds should all be mixed in a jar or other container.
2. Mix thoroughly to blend.
3. For at least four hrs, preferably overnight, cover and chill.
4. Stir one more in the morning, and if preferred, add honey or maple syrup.
5. Present chilled.

Nutrition Info (per serving):

Calories: 220

Protein: 6g

Carbs: 45g

Fat: 4g

Fiber: 8g

Prep Time: 10 min

Cook Time: 0 min

Servings: 1

Points Values: 5 per serving

Ingredients:

- 1 cup of unsweetened almond milk
- 1 scoop vanilla protein powder
- 1/2 cup of frozen berries
- 1/2 banana
- 1 tbsp chia seeds
- 1/4 cup of granola
- Fresh berries and split banana for topping

Instructions:

1. Blend protein powder, frozen berries, banana, chia seeds, and almond milk in a blender. Process till smooth.
2. Transfer the smoothie to a bowl.
3. Add granola, banana slices, and fresh berries over top.
4. Serve right away.

Nutrition Info (per serving):

Calories: 280

Protein: 20g

Carbs: 42g

Fat: 7g

Fiber: 9g

Prep Time: 10 min

Cook Time: 20 min

Servings: 2

Points Values: 6 per serving

Ingredients:

- One large sweet potato that has been peeled and diced
- 1/2 cup of black beans, drained and rinsed
- 1/2 red bell pepper, diced
- 1/2 onion, diced
- 2 cloves garlic, minced
- 1 tbsp olive oil
- 1 tsp ground cumin
- 1 tsp paprika
- Salt and pepper to taste
- 2 large eggs (non-compulsory)

Instructions:

1. In a big skillet over medium heat, warm up the olive oil.
2. Add the sweet potato and simmer for about ten min, or until it begins to soften.
3. Add the garlic, onion, and bell pepper. Simmer the veggies for 5 min or until they are soft.
4. Add the paprika, cumin, black beans, salt, and pepper and stir. Cook until well cooked, 2 to 3 min more.
5. If you're serving eggs with the hash, cook them to your desired doneness in a different pan.
6. Serve right away.

Nutrition Info (per serving without eggs):

Calories: 250

Protein: 6g

Carbs: 45g

Fat: 8g Fiber: 10g

Prep Time: 10 min

Cook Time: 10 min

Servings: 4

Points Values: 5 per serving

Ingredients:

- 4 whole wheat tortillas
- 4 large eggs
- 4 large egg whites
- 1/2 cup of black beans, drained and rinsed
- 1/2 cup of salsa
- 1/2 cup of low-fat cheddar cheese that has been shredded
- 1/4 cup of chop-up cilantro
- Cooking spray

Instructions:

1. The eggs and egg whites should be whisked together in a basin.
2. Apply cooking spray to a nonstick skillet and heat it over medium heat.
3. Add the eggs and heat, stirring now and then, until well cooked and scrambled.
4. Toast tortillas or reheat them in the microwave.
5. Among the tortillas, distribute equally the eggs, black beans, salsa, cheese, and cilantro.
6. To make burritos, roll up your tortillas.
7. Serve right away.

Nutrition Info (per serving):

Calories: 280

Protein: 20g

Carbs: 34g

Fat: 9g

Fiber: 8g

Prep Time: 10 min

Cook Time: 15 min

Servings: 2

Points Values: 6 per serving

Ingredients:

- 1/2 cup of quinoa
- 1 cup of water
- 1 avocado, diced
- 1/2 cup of cherry tomatoes, halved
- 2 large eggs
- 2 tbsp crumbled feta cheese
- Salt and pepper to taste
- 1 tbsp olive oil

Instructions:

1. Wash the quinoa in cool water.
2. Add water to the quinoa in a saucepan. After bringing to a boil, lower the heat to a simmer for fifteen min, or until all of the water has been absorbed.
3. In the meantime, fry eggs to your preference in a skillet with medium-high heat and olive oil.
4. Spoon cooked quinoa into every of two bowls.
5. Add cooked eggs, feta cheese, cherry tomatoes, and cubed avocado to the top of every bowl.
6. Toss in some salt and pepper and season to taste.
7. Serve right away.

Nutrition Info (per serving):

Calories: 350

Protein: 13g

Carbs: 32g

Fat: 21g

Fiber: 8g

Prep Time: 10 min

Cook Time: 10 min

Servings: 4 (2 waffles per serving)

Points Values: 6 per serving

Ingredients:

- 1 cup of whole wheat flour
- 1 tbsp baking powder
- 1 tbsp sugar
- 1/4 tsp salt
- 1 cup of unsweetened almond milk
- 2 large eggs
- 2 tbsp melted coconut oil
- 1 tsp vanilla extract
- Fresh fruit (berries, banana slices) for topping

Instructions:

1. Warm up the waffle maker.
2. Mix the flour, baking powder, sugar, and salt in a big bowl.
3. Whisk together the eggs, melted coconut oil, almond milk, and vanilla extract in a separate bowl.
4. Mix the dry ingredients with the wet ones until they are barely mixed.
5. After the waffle iron has heated up, pour the batter into it and fry it as directed by the maker until it turns golden brown.
6. Add some fresh fruit on top and serve right away.

Nutrition Info (per serving):

Calories: 280

Protein: 9g

Carbs: 36g

Fat: 12g

Fiber: 6g

Prep Time: 5 min

Cook Time: 5 min

Servings: 1

Points Values: 5 per serving

Ingredients:

- 1 slice whole grain bread, toasted
- 1/2 avocado, mashed
- 1 large egg
- 1 tsp lemon juice
- Salt and pepper to taste
- Red pepper flakes (non-compulsory)

Instructions:

1. Heat a small saucepan of water until it gently simmers.
2. Break the egg into a little basin. Simmer the water until it forms a moderate vortex, then slip the egg into the center. Cook for three to four min, or until the yolk is still runny and the white is set.
3. Spread mashed avocado on the toast while the egg poaches. Sprinkle with salt and pepper and drizzle with lemon juice.
4. Using a slotted spoon, carefully remove the poached egg and set it on top of the avocado toast.
5. If preferred, top with red pepper flakes and serve right away.

Nutrition Info (per serving):

Calories: 250

Protein: 10g

Carbs: 24g

Fat: 14g

Fiber: 7g

Prep Time: 10 min

Cook Time: 10 min

Servings: 4

Points Values: 5 per serving

Ingredients:

- 4 toasted and split whole wheat English muffins
- 4 lean turkey sausage patties
- 4 large eggs
- 4 slices reduced-fat cheddar cheese
- Cooking spray

Instructions:

1. Apply cooking spray to a nonstick skillet and heat it over medium heat.
2. Cook for 4–5 min on every side, or until turkey sausage patties are thoroughly cooked and browned.
3. Cook eggs according as needed in a different pan.
4. Place a sausage patty, a cheese slice, and an egg on either half of an English muffin to assemble the sandwiches.
5. Serve right away.

Nutrition Info (per serving):

Calories: 300

Protein: 25g

Carbs: 30g

Fat: 10g

Fiber: 5g

Prep Time: 5 min

Cook Time: 0 min

Servings: 1

Points Values: 4 per serving

Ingredients:

- 1 banana
- 1 tbsp natural peanut butter
- 1 cup of unsweetened almond milk
- 1/2 cup onion-fat Greek yogurt
- 1 tsp honey (non-compulsory)
- Ice cubes (non-compulsory)

Instructions:

1. Mix all ingredients in a blender.
2. Blend until smooth.
3. Serve immediately.

Nutrition Info (per serving):

Calories: 250

Protein: 12g

Carbs: 35g

Fat: 8g

Fiber: 4g

Prep Time: 5 min

Cook Time: 0 min

Servings: 1

Points Values: 3 per serving

Ingredients:

- 1 cup of low-fat cottage cheese
- 1/2 cup of mixed fresh fruit
- 1 tsp honey
- 1 tbsp chop-up nuts (non-compulsory)

Instructions:

1. Mix the mixed fruit and cottage cheese in a bowl.
2. Pour some honey over it.
3. If desired, top with chop-up nuts.
4. Serve right away.

Nutrition Info (per serving):

Calories: 180

Protein: 14g

Carbs: 22g

Fat: 4g

Fiber: 2g

Prep Time: 15 min

Cook Time: 25 min

Servings: 12 muffins

Points Values: 3 per serving

Ingredients:

- 1 1/2 cups of finely grated zucchini (about 2 medium)
- 1 cup of whole wheat flour
- 1/2 cup of all-purpose flour
- 1 tsp baking powder
- 1/2 tsp baking soda
- 1/2 tsp salt
- 1/2 tsp garlic powder
- 1/2 tsp onion powder
- 1/2 cup of low-fat cheddar cheese that has been shredded
- 1/4 cup of finely grated Parmesan cheese
- 1/4 cup of plain Greek yogurt
- 2 large eggs
- 1/4 cup of olive oil

Instructions:

1. Turn the oven on to 350°F. Use paper liners and cooking spray to line a muffin tray.
2. Mix the flour, baking soda, baking powder, salt, onion powder, and garlic powder in a big bowl.
3. Whisk together eggs, Greek yogurt, and olive oil in a separate bowl.
4. Just mix the wet and dry ingredients by stirring them together. Stir in cheeses and zucchini.
5. Evenly distribute the batter among the muffin liners.
6. When a toothpick put into the center comes out clean, bake for 20 to 25 min.
7. Let cool somewhat before arranging to serve.

Nutrition Info (per serving):

Calories: 130

Protein: 5g Carbs: 12g Fat: 7g Fiber: 2g

GRILLED CHICKEN AND MANGO SALAD

Prep Time: 15 min

Cook Time: 15 min

Servings: 4

Points Values: 6 per serving

Ingredients:

- 2 boneless, skinless chicken breasts
- 1 ripe mango, diced
- 6 cups of mixed salad greens
- 1/4 cup of split almonds
- 1/4 cup of diced red onion
- 1/4 cup of crumbled feta cheese
- 2 tbsp balsamic vinaigrette dressing

Instructions:

1. Grill at a medium-high temperature.
2. Add salt and pepper to chicken breasts for seasoning.
3. Cook the chicken for 6–7 minutes on every side, or until it's thoroughly cooked. Slice after letting cool slightly.
4. Mix the chop-up mango, split almonds, red onion, crumbled feta cheese, and mixed greens in a big bowl.
5. Add a balsamic vinaigrette dressing to the salad.
6. Arrange salad into plates, then add slices of cooked chicken on top.
7. Serve right away.

Nutrition Info (per serving):

Calories: 290

Protein: 26g

Carbohydrates: 18g

Fat: 12g Fiber: 5g

Prep Time: 15 min

Cook Time: 10 min

Servings: 4

Points Values: 4 per serving

Ingredients:

- 1 lb ground turkey
- 1 tbsp olive oil
- 1 tsp garlic powder
- 1 tsp onion powder
- Salt and pepper to taste
- 1 avocado, split
- 1 cup of diced tomatoes
- 1/2 cup of diced red onion
- 1/4 cup of chop-up cilantro
- 8 large lettuce leaves

Instructions:

1. The olive oil should be warmed in a skillet set over medium heat.
2. Add the onion, garlic, and powdered turkey along with the salt and pepper. Break up the turkey with a spoon while it cooks and continue to cook until it is browned and cooked through.
3. Diced tomatoes, diced red onion, and chopped-up cilantro should all be mixed in a bowl.
4. Spoon cooked turkey onto every lettuce leaf to assemble the wraps.
5. Add tomato salsa and split avocado on top.
6. Serve lettuce right away after rolling the leaves.

Nutrition Info (per serving):

Calories: 270

Protein: 21g

Carbohydrates: 12g

Fat: 16g Fiber: 5g

Prep Time: 20 min

Cook Time: 35 min

Servings: 4

Points Values: 6 per serving

Ingredients:

- 4 large bell peppers
- 1 cup of cooked quinoa
- 1 cup of black beans, drained and rinsed
- 1 cup of corn kernels
- 1 cup of diced tomatoes
- 1/2 cup of diced red onion
- 1/4 cup of chop-up cilantro
- 1 tsp ground cumin
- 1 tsp chili powder
- Salt and pepper to taste
- 1/2 cup of low-fat cheddar cheese that has been shredded (non-compulsory)

Instructions:

1. Turn the oven on to 375°F. Cut off the bell peppers' tops to extract the seeds and membranes.
2. Cooked quinoa, black beans, corn, chopped tomatoes, red onion, cilantro, ground cumin, chili powder, salt, and pepper should all be mixed in a big bowl.
3. Fill every bell pepper to the brim with the quinoa mixture.
4. Cover the filled peppers with foil after placing them in a roasting dish.
5. Bake peppers for 25 to 30 min, or until soft.
6. Remove the foil, top the peppers with the shredded cheddar cheese, if using, and bake for a further five min, or until the cheese is melted.
7. Warm up the food.

Nutrition Info (per serving):

Calories: 310

Protein: 16g

Carbohydrates: 49g Fat: 6g Fiber: 12g

Prep Time: 15 min

Cook Time: 0 min

Servings: 4

Points Values: 5 per serving

Ingredients:

- 2 cups of cooked chickpeas
- 1 cup of diced cucumber
- 1 cup of cherry tomatoes, halved
- 1/2 cup of diced red onion
- 1/4 cup of chop-up Kalamata olives
- 1/4 cup of crumbled feta cheese
- 2 tbsp chop-up fresh parsley
- 2 tbsp extra virgin olive oil
- 1 tbsp lemon juice
- 1 tsp dried oregano
- Salt and pepper to taste

Instructions:

1. Cooked chickpeas, split cucumber, cherry tomatoes, red onion, feta cheese, Kalamata olives, and parsley should all be mixed in a big bowl.
2. Mix the extra virgin olive oil, lemon juice, dried oregano, salt, and pepper in a small bowl.
3. Drizzle the chickpea salad with the dressing and mix thoroughly.
4. Serve right away or put in the fridge until you're ready to serve.

Nutrition Info (per serving):

Calories: 290

Protein: 11g

Carbohydrates: 25g

Fat: 16g

Fiber: 7g

Prep Time: 15 min

Cook Time: 0 min

Servings: 4

Points Values: 7 per serving

Ingredients:

- 4 whole wheat tortillas
- 2 cups of chicken breast that has been cooked and shredded
- 1 cup of chop-up romaine lettuce
- 1/4 cup of finely grated Parmesan cheese
- 1/4 cup of light Caesar dressing
- Salt and pepper to taste

Instructions:

1. Divide the shredded chicken evenly among the tortillas that have been laid out.
2. Add a little Caesar dressing, finely grated Parmesan cheese, and chop-up romaine lettuce to the chicken.
3. Toss in some salt and pepper and season to taste.
4. Tighten tortillas into wraps, if necessary, using toothpicks.
5. Serve right away.

Nutrition Info (per serving):

Calories: 280

Protein: 24g

Carbohydrates: 23g

Fat: 10g

Fiber: 4g

Prep Time: 20 min

Cook Time: 10 min

Servings: 4

Points Values: 6 per serving

Ingredients:

- One pound of large shrimp, deveined and shell-free
- 2 tsp chili powder
- 1 tsp ground cumin
- 1/2 tsp garlic powder
- 1/2 tsp onion powder
- Salt and pepper to taste
- 1 mango, diced
- 1/2 red onion, lightly chop-up
- 1 jalapeno, seeded and minced
- 1/4 cup of chop-up fresh cilantro
- Juice of 1 lime
- 8 small corn tortillas
- 1 cup of shredded cabbage
- 1 avocado, split

Instructions:

1. Mix the onion, garlic, and chili powders, cumin, salt, and pepper in a bowl and toss to cover the shrimp evenly.
2. In a skillet, preheat the heat to medium-high. Stir in shrimp and cook for 2 to 3 min on every side, or until cooked through and pink.
3. To create the salsa, mix the diced mango, chop-upjalapeño, chop-up red onion, cilantro, and lime juice in a separate bowl.
4. Corn tortillas can be reheated in a microwave or dry skillet.
5. Place shrimp on every tortilla, then top with avocado slices, shredded cabbage, and mango salsa to assemble the tacos.
6. Serve right away.

Nutrition Info (per serving):

Calories: 320 Protein: 24g Carbohydrates: 34g Fat: 12g Fiber: 7g

Prep Time: 15 min

Cook Time: 35 min

Servings: 6

Points Values: 4 per serving

Ingredients:

- 1 cup of dried green lentils
- 1 onion, diced
- 2 carrots, diced
- 2 celery stalks, diced
- 2 garlic cloves, minced
- 6 cups of vegetable broth
- 1 can (14 oz) diced tomatoes
- 1 tsp dried thyme
- 1 tsp dried oregano
- Salt and pepper to taste
- Fresh parsley, chop-up (for garnish)

Instructions:

1. After rinsing with cold water, drain the lentils.
2. The vegetable broth should be heated to a boil in a large saucepan over medium heat. Add the chop-up celery, carrots, onion, and garlic. Simmer the veggies for 5 min or until they are tender.
3. To the pot, add the lentils, diced tomatoes, oregano, thyme, and salt and pepper. Once the lentils are soft, decrease the heat to low and simmer for 25 to 30 min after bringing them to a boil.
4. Taste and adjust the seasoning.
5. If desired, top a hot dish with chop-up parsley.

Nutrition Info (per serving):

Calories: 220

Protein: 13g

Carbohydrates: 40g

Fat: 1g Fiber: 9g

Prep Time: 20 min

Cook Time: 15 min

Servings: 4

Points Values: 5 per serving

Ingredients:

- 1 lb boneless, skinless chicken breasts, thinly split
- 2 tbsp Greek yogurt
- 1 tbsp lemon juice
- 1 tsp dried oregano
- 1 clove garlic, minced
- Salt and pepper to taste
- 4 whole wheat pita breads
- 1 cup of diced cucumber
- 1 cup of diced tomatoes
- 1/2 cup of diced red onion
- 1/4 cup of chop-up fresh parsley
- Tzatziki sauce for serving (non-compulsory)

Instructions:

1. Greek yogurt, lemon juice, chopped garlic, dried oregano, salt, and pepper should all be mixed with thinly split chicken breasts in a bowl. For at least fifteen min, marinate.
2. In a skillet, preheat the heat to medium-high. After adding the marinated chicken slices, grill them for 5 to 6 min on every side, or until done.
3. Warm up whole wheat pita bread in the microwave or on a dry skillet.
4. Place cooked chicken slices, diced tomatoes, split red onion, and diced cucumber, and chop up fresh parsley inside every pita pocket.
5. If desired, drizzle with tzatziki sauce.
6. Serve right away.

Nutrition Info (per serving):

Calories: 310

Protein: 30g Carbohydrates: 30g Fat: 8g Fiber: 5g

Prep Time: 15 min

Cook Time: 15 min

Servings: 4

Points Values: 5 per serving

Ingredients:

- 1 lb ground turkey
- 1 tbsp sesame oil
- 2 cloves garlic, minced
- 1 tbsp fresh ginger, minced
- 1/4 cup of soy sauce
- 2 tbsp hoisin sauce
- 1 tbsp rice vinegar
- 1 tsp sriracha sauce (non-compulsory)
- 1 cup of shredded carrots
- 1/2 cup of split water chestnuts, drained
- 1/4 cup of chop-up green onions
- 1 head butter lettuce, leaves separated

Instructions:

1. In a big skillet, warm up the sesame oil over medium-high heat.
2. Add the ginger, garlic, and ground turkey. Break up the turkey with a spoon and sauté until it's browned and cooked through.
3. Mix the rice vinegar, sriracha sauce, hoisin sauce, and soy sauce in a small bowl.
4. Cover the cooked turkey in the skillet with sauce. Add the water chestnuts and shredded carrots. After combining, cook for an additional two to three min.
5. After taking off the heat, add the chop-up green onions.
6. Spoon the turkey mixture into every lettuce leaf as a serving dish.
7. Serve right away.

Nutrition Info (per serving):

Calories: 280

Protein: 25g

Carbohydrates: 11g Fat: 15g Fiber: 3g

Prep Time: 10 min

Cook Time: 0 min

Servings: 2

Points Values: 4 per serving

Ingredients:

- 2 large whole wheat tortillas
- 1/2 cup of hummus
- 1 cup of mixed salad greens
- 1/2 cup of shredded carrots
- 1/2 cup of split cucumbers
- 1/2 cup of split bell peppers
- 1/4 cup of split red onion
- 1/4 cup of crumbled feta cheese (non-compulsory)

Instructions:

1. After arranging the tortillas, top everyone with 1/4 cup of hummus.
2. Spoon shredded carrots, split bell peppers, split red onion, split cucumbers, and mixed salad greens between every one of the two tortillas.
3. Top the vegetables with crumbled feta cheese, if using.
4. Tortillas are rolled into wraps.
5. Cut wraps in half, then serve right away.

Nutrition Info (per serving):

Calories: 320

Protein: 10g

Carbohydrates: 42g

Fat: 14g

Fiber: 10g

Prep Time: 10 min

Cook Time: 15 min

Servings: 4

Points Values: 6 per serving

Ingredients:

- 4 salmon fillets
- Salt and pepper to taste
- 1 lb asparagus, ends trimmed
- 2 tbsp olive oil
- 1/4 cup of balsamic vinegar
- 2 tbsp honey
- 2 cloves garlic, minced
- 1 tsp dried thyme
- Lemon wedges for serving

Instructions:

1. Turn the oven on to 400°F.
2. Use salt and pepper to season the salmon fillets. Transfer them to a parchment paper-lined baking sheet.
3. Add salt, pepper, and olive oil to the chop-up asparagus and toss. Place them on the baking sheet around the salmon.
4. Balsamic vinegar, honey, chopped garlic, and dried thyme should all be mixed in a small saucepan. Over medium heat, bring to a simmer and cook for 3–4 min, or until slightly thickened.
5. Drizzle the salmon fillets with half of the balsamic glaze.
6. For 12 to 15 min, or until the salmon is cooked through and flaked easily with a fork, roast the asparagus together with the salmon in the preheated oven.
7. Take the salmon out of the oven and drizzle the leftover balsamic glaze over it.
8. Warm-up and accompany with wedges of lemon.

Nutrition Info (per serving):

Calories: 350

Protein: 25g Carbohydrates: 17g Fat: 20g Fiber: 3g

Prep Time: 15 min

Cook Time: 0 min

Servings: 4

Points Values: 3 per serving

Ingredients:

- 4 medium zucchinis
- 1 cup of cherry tomatoes, halved
- 3/4 cup of halved fresh mozzarella balls
- 1/4 cup of chop-up fresh basil
- 2 tbsp extra virgin olive oil
- 2 tbsp balsamic vinegar
- Salt and pepper to taste

Instructions:

1. Spiralize the zucchini to make noodles with a spiralizer.
2. Mix the chop-up fresh basil, cherry tomatoes, fresh mozzarella balls, and zucchini noodles in a big bowl.
3. Over the salad, drizzle some extra virgin olive oil and balsamic vinegar.
4. Toss in some salt and pepper and season to taste.
5. Gently toss to mix.
6. Serve right away and put in the fridge until you're ready to serve.

Nutrition Info (per serving):

Calories: 150

Protein: 6g

Carbohydrates: 8g

Fat: 11g

Fiber: 2g

Prep Time: 15 min

Cook Time: 4 hrs on High or 8 hrs on Low

Servings: 6

Points Values: 6 per serving

Ingredients:

- 1 lb boneless, skinless chicken breasts
- 1 can (15 oz) diced tomatoes
- 1 can (4 oz) diced green chilies
- 1 onion, diced
- 1 bell pepper, diced
- 2 cloves garlic, minced
- 4 cups of low-sodium chicken broth
- 1 cup of frozen corn kernels
- 1 tsp chili powder
- 1 tsp ground cumin
- 1/2 tsp smoked paprika
- Salt and pepper to taste
- Tortilla strips, avocado slices, shredded cheese, and chop-up cilantro for serving

Instructions:

1. In a slow cooker, place the chicken breasts.
2. Put frozen corn kernels, diced tomatoes, diced green chilies, diced onion, diced bell pepper, chop-up garlic, chicken stock, smoked paprika, cumin, and chili powder in the slow cooker.
3. Once the chicken is thoroughly cooked and tender, cover and simmer it for 4 hrs on High or 8 hrs on Low.
4. Take the chicken out of the slow cooker and use two forks to shred it. Add the chicken shreds back to the slow cooker and mix everything.
5. Top with avocado slices, chop-up cilantro, shredded cheese, and tortilla strips, and serve hot.

Nutrition Info (per serving):

Calories: 240

Protein: 25g Carbohydrates: 21g Fat: 6g Fiber: 4g

Prep Time: 15 min

Cook Time: 20 min

Servings: 4

Points Values: 5 per serving

Ingredients:

- 1 cup of quinoa, rinsed
- 2 cups of water
- 1/4 cup of raisins
- 1/4 cup of chop-up dried apricots
- 1/4 cup of chop-up almonds
- 1/4 cup of chop-up fresh parsley
- 1/4 cup of chop-up fresh cilantro
- 2 tbsp olive oil
- 1 tbsp lemon juice
- 1 tsp ground cumin
- 1/2 tsp ground cinnamon
- 1/2 tsp ground ginger
- Salt and pepper to taste
- Non-compulsory: split green onions for garnish

Instructions:

1. Bring water or vegetable broth to a boil in a medium-sized saucepan. Lower the heat to low and stir in the quinoa. After the quinoa is cooked and the water has been absorbed, cover and simmer for 15 to 20 min.
2. Cooked quinoa, raisins, chop-up almonds, chop-up dried apricots, chop-up fresh parsley, and chop-up fresh cilantro should all be mixed in a big bowl.
3. Mix the olive oil, lemon juice, ground ginger, cinnamon, cumin, and salt & pepper in a small bowl.
4. Drizzle the quinoa mixture with the dressing and mix thoroughly.
5. If preferred, top cold with chop-up green onions.

Nutrition Info (per serving):

Calories: 310

Protein: 8g Carbohydrates: 42g Fat: 13g Fiber: 6g

Prep Time: 10 min

Cook Time: 0 min

Servings: 4

Points Values: 3 per serving

Ingredients:

- 2 cans (5 oz every) tuna, drained
- 1 can (15 oz) white beans, drained and rinsed
- 1/2 red onion, lightly chop-up
- 1/4 cup of chop-up fresh parsley
- 2 tbsp olive oil
- 2 tbsp lemon juice
- 1 tsp Dijon mustard
- Salt and pepper to taste
- Non-compulsory: cherry tomatoes, cucumber slices, and mixed salad greens for serving

Instructions:

1. Drained tuna, rinsed and drained white beans, lightly chopped up red onion, and chopped fresh parsley should all be mixed in a big bowl.
2. To create the dressing, mix the olive oil, lemon juice, Dijon mustard, salt, and pepper in a small bowl.
3. Drizzle the tuna and white bean mixture with the dressing. Lightly coat all things by tossing.
4. Serve right away either this way or, if preferred, over a bed of mixed salad greens with cherry tomatoes and cucumber slices as garnish.

Nutrition Info (per serving):

Calories: 250

Protein: 22g

Carbohydrates: 21g

Fat: 9g

Fiber: 6g

LEMON HERB GRILLED CHICKEN WITH QUINOA

Prep Time: 10 min

Cook Time: 15 min

Servings: 4

Points Values: 6 per serving

Ingredients:

- 4 boneless, skinless chicken breasts
- Zest and juice of 1 lemon
- 2 cloves garlic, minced
- 1 tbsp chop-up fresh parsley
- 1 tbsp chop-up fresh thyme
- 2 tbsp olive oil
- Salt and pepper to taste
- 1 cup of quinoa
- 2 cups of chicken broth

Instructions:

1. Lemon zest, lemon juice, chop-up garlic, chop-up parsley, chop-up thyme, olive oil, salt, and pepper should all be mixed in a bowl.
2. Coat the chicken breasts uniformly by placing them in the marinade. Allow to marinate in the refrigerator for at least 30 min or overnight.
3. Grill at a medium-high temperature. Chicken breasts should be cooked through and no longer pink in the center after grilling them for 6–7 min on every side.
4. Rinse and drain the quinoa under cold water while the chicken is grilling. Bring water or chicken broth to a boil in a saucepan. When the quinoa is cooked and the liquid has been absorbed, add it, lower the heat to low, cover it, and simmer for 15 min.
5. Serve cooked quinoa alongside grilled chicken.

Nutrition Info (per serving):

Calories: 380

Protein: 34g Carbohydrates: 25g Fat: 14g Fiber: 3g

Prep Time: 15 min

Cook Time: 1 hr 15 min

Servings: 4

Points Values: 5 per serving

Ingredients:

- 1 medium spaghetti squash
- 1 lb lean ground beef or turkey
- 1 onion, diced
- 2 cloves garlic, minced
- 1 carrot, finely grated
- 1 celery stalk, diced
- 1 can (14 oz) crushed tomatoes
- 1/4 cup of tomato paste
- 1/2 cup of beef
- 1 tbsp olive oil
- 1 tsp dried oregano
- 1 tsp dried basil
- Salt and pepper to taste
- Finely grated Parmesan cheese for serving (non-compulsory)

Instructions:

1. Turn the oven on to 400°F. After cutting the spaghetti squash in half lengthwise, remove the seeds.
2. Halve the squash and place the cut side down on a parchment paper-lined baking sheet. Bake the squash for 45 to 50 min, or until it is fork-tender.
3. Heat the olive oil in a big skillet over medium heat while the squash bakes. Add the diced celery, finely grated carrot, chopped-up garlic, and onion. Simmer the veggies for 5 min or until they are tender.
4. Pour ground turkey or beef into the skillet. Break it up with a spoon while it cooks until it's browned and cooked through.
5. Add the tomato paste, crushed tomatoes, dried basil, dried oregano, beef or vegetable broth, salt, and pepper. Simmer the sauce for 15 to 20 min, or until it thickens.
6. After the spaghetti squash is cooked, scrape the meat into spaghetti-like strands with a fork.
7. Top spaghetti squash with Bolognese sauce and serve. If preferred, top with finely grated Parmesan cheese.

Nutrition Info (per serving):

Calories: 320 Protein: 26g Carbohydrates: 24g Fat: 12g Fiber: 6g

Prep Time: 10 min

Cook Time: 20 min

Servings: 4

Points Values: 7 per serving

Ingredients:

- 4 salmon fillets
- 1 lb baby potatoes, halved
- 2 cups of broccoli florets
- 1 bell pepper, split
- 1 zucchini, split
- 2 tbsp olive oil
- 2 cloves garlic, minced
- 1 tsp dried thyme
- 1 tsp dried rosemary
- Salt and pepper to taste
- Lemon wedges for serving

Instructions:

1. Turn the oven on to 400°F. Line a baking sheet with parchment paper.
2. Mix olive oil, chop-up garlic, dried thyme, dried rosemary, salt, and pepper in a big bowl and stir with halved baby potatoes, broccoli florets, split bell pepper, and split zucchini.
3. Arrange the vegetables on the prepared baking sheet in a single layer. Roast for ten min in the preheated oven.
4. After taking the baking sheet out of the oven, arrange the partially roasted veggies on top of the salmon fillets. Sear the salmon with a little salt and pepper.
5. Place the baking sheet back in the oven and roast for an additional ten min, or until the veggies are soft and the salmon is cooked through.
6. Serve hot with wedges of lemon.

Nutrition Info (per serving):

Calories: 380

Protein: 30g Carbohydrates: 20g Fat: 20g Fiber: 5g

Prep Time: 15 min

Cook Time: 15 min

Servings: 4

Points Values: 4 per serving

Ingredients:

- 1 lb lean ground turkey
- 2 tbsp soy sauce
- 1 tbsp oyster sauce
- 1 tbsp sesame oil
- 1 tbsp cornstarch
- 1 onion, split
- 2 bell peppers, split
- 1 cup of split mushrooms
- 1 cup of snap peas
- 2 cloves garlic, minced
- Cooked brown rice for serving

Instructions:

1. Mix the soy sauce, oyster sauce, sesame oil, and cornstarch in a small bowl. Put aside.
2. A big wok or skillet should be heated to medium-high heat. Break up the ground turkey with a spoon while it cooks until it turns brown.
3. To the skillet, add the diced onion, bell peppers, mushrooms, snap peas, and chopped-up garlic. Stir-fry the vegetables for 5 to 7 min, or until they are crisp-tender.
4. Cover the turkey and vegetables with the sauce mixture. Cook, stirring, for a further two to three min, or until the sauce has thickened.
5. Overcooked brown rice, served hot.

Nutrition Info (per serving):

Calories: 280

Protein: 24g

Carbohydrates: 20g Fat: 10g Fiber: 4g

Prep Time: 20 min

Cook Time: 30 min

Servings: 4

Points Values: 6 per serving

Ingredients:

- 1 large eggplant, split into 1/2-inch rounds
- Salt
- 1 cup of breadcrumbs
- 1/2 cup of finely grated Parmesan cheese
- 2 eggs, beaten
- 1 cup of marinara sauce
- 1 cup of shredded mozzarella cheese
- Fresh basil leaves for garnish (non-compulsory)

Instructions:

1. Set oven temperature to 400°F. A baking sheet can be lined with parchment paper or greased.
2. Arrange the slices of eggplant on a baking sheet covered with paper towels. To relieve excess moisture, sprinkle them with salt and leave them for approximately fifteen min. Using a different paper towel, pat dry.
3. Finely grated Parmesan cheese and breadcrumbs should be mixed in a shallow plate.
4. Beat the eggs in a different shallow dish.
5. After dipping every eggplant slice into the beaten eggs, lightly press the breadcrumb mixture onto it to ensure it adheres. Spoon the coated slices onto the ready baking sheet.
6. Bake for 15 to 20 min, or until the eggplant slices are crispy and golden brown, in a preheated oven.
7. Take out of the oven the baking sheet. Every eggplant slice should have a thin coating of marinara sauce applied to it, followed by shredded mozzarella cheese.
8. Put the baking sheet back in the oven and continue baking for ten more min, or until the cheese is bubbling and melted.
9. If preferred, top with freshly chopped-up basil leaves and serve hot.

Nutrition Info (per serving):

Calories: 320

Protein: 18g

Carbohydrates: 25g Fat: 16g Fiber: 5g

Prep Time: 15 min

Cook Time: 4 hrs on Low

Servings: 6

Points Values: 8 per serving

Ingredients:

- 1 1/2 lbs flank steak, thinly split
- 1 cup of beef broth
- 1/2 cup of low-sodium soy sauce
- 1/3 cup of brown sugar
- 1 tbsp sesame oil
- 3 cloves garlic, minced
- 2 tbsp cornstarch
- 2 tbsp water
- 4 cups of broccoli florets
- Cooked rice

Instructions:

1. Add the chopped garlic, brown sugar, sesame oil, soy sauce, and beef broth to the slow cooker. Mix thoroughly until fully incorporated.
2. Toss the thinly split flank steak in the sauce after adding it to the slow cooker.
3. Cook for 4 hrs on Low with a cover on.
4. Make a slurry by combining cornstarch and water in a small bowl. To thicken the sauce in the last half hour of cooking, stir the slurry into the slow cooker.
5. For the final thirty min of simmering, add broccoli florets to the slow cooker. Mix everything.
6. On cooked rice, serve the beef and broccoli.

Nutrition Info (per serving):

Calories: 320

Protein: 26g

Carbohydrates: 23g

Fat: 12g Fiber: 3g

Prep Time: 10 min

Cook Time: 25 min

Servings: 4

Points Values: 5 per serving

Ingredients:

- 1 lb pork tenderloin
- 2 tbsp Dijon mustard
- 1 tbsp olive oil
- 1 tbsp chop-up fresh thyme
- 1 tbsp chop-up fresh rosemary
- 1 tbsp chop-up fresh parsley
- Salt and pepper to taste

Instructions:

1. Turn the oven on to 425°F.
2. To make a paste, mix the Dijon mustard, olive oil, chop-up parsley, chop-up rosemary, chop-up thyme, and salt & pepper in a small bowl.
3. Evenly coat the pork tenderloin by rubbing it with the herb paste.
4. Arrange the pork tenderloin onto a parchment paper-lined baking sheet.
5. For medium doneness, roast in the preheated oven for 20 to 25 min, or until the internal temperature reaches 145°F.
6. Before slicing, take the pork tenderloin out of the oven and allow it to rest for five min.
7. After slicing, serve the pork tenderloin.

Nutrition Info (per serving):

Calories: 280

Protein: 30g

Carbohydrates: 1g

Fat: 16g

Fiber: 0g

Prep Time: 20 min

Cook Time: 25 min

Servings: 4

Points Values: 6 per serving

Ingredients:

- 1 head cauliflower, riced
- 1 egg
- 1/2 cup of shredded mozzarella cheese
- 1/4 cup of finely grated Parmesan cheese
- 1 tsp dried oregano
- 1 tsp dried basil
- Salt and pepper to taste
- 1/2 cup of marinara sauce
- 1/2 cup of shredded mozzarella cheese
- Fresh basil leaves
- Split tomatoes

Instructions:

1. Turn the oven on to 425°F. Line a baking sheet with parchment paper.
2. Heat the riced cauliflower in a microwave-safe bowl for five to six min, or until it becomes soft. Allow it to cool a little.
3. After cooking, transfer the cauliflower to a fresh cheesecloth or dish towel and squeeze out as much moisture as you can.
4. The cauliflower, egg, finely grated Parmesan cheese, dried oregano, dried basil, salt, and pepper should all be mixed in a mixing dish. Blend until thoroughly blended.
5. Forming the cauliflower mixture into a circle, press it onto the baking sheet that has been preheated to create the pizza crust.
6. In a preheated oven, bake the cauliflower crust for 15 to 18 min, or until it sets and turns golden brown.
7. After taking the cauliflower crust out of the oven, cover it with marinara sauce. Disperse the shredded mozzarella cheese over the sauce.
8. Top the cheese with split tomatoes and fresh basil leaves.
9. Put the pizza back in the oven and continue to bake it for a further 8 to 10 min, or until the cheese is bubbling and melted.
10. Serve the Margherita pizza with a split cauliflower crust.

Nutrition Info (per serving):

Calories: 200 Protein: 12g Carbohydrates: 10g Fat: 12g Fiber: 4g

Prep Time: 15 min

Cook Time: 10 min

Servings: 4

Points Values: 3 per serving

Ingredients:

- One pound of large shrimp, deveined and shell-free
- Salt and pepper to taste
- 2 tbsp olive oil
- 4 cloves garlic, minced
- Zest and juice of 1 lemon
- 4 medium zucchinis, spiralized into zoodles
- Chop-up fresh parsley for garnish

Instructions:

1. To taste, add salt and pepper to the shrimp to season them.
2. In a big skillet set over medium-high heat, warm up the olive oil. Add the chopped garlic and simmer for one minute, or until fragrant.
3. When the shrimp are opaque and pink, add them to the skillet and cook for two to three min on every side.
4. Juice and zest the lemon, then whisk in.
5. In the skillet, add the spiralized zucchini and mix with the shrimp and garlic lemon sauce. Heat for two min, or until the zucchini is slightly softened.
6. Before serving, remove from the heat and sprinkle with freshly cut parsley.

Nutrition Info (per serving):

Calories: 180

Protein: 25g

Carbohydrates: 6g

Fat: 8g

Fiber: 2g

Prep Time: 15 min

Cook Time: 1 hr 15 min

Servings: 4

Points Values: 7 per serving

Ingredients:

- 1 lb boneless, skinless chicken thighs, cut into bite-sized pieces
- 2 tbsp olive oil
- 1 onion, diced
- 2 cloves garlic, minced
- 1 tsp ground cumin
- 1 tsp ground coriander
- 1/2 tsp ground cinnamon
- 1/2 tsp ground ginger
- 1/4 tsp ground turmeric
- 1/4 tsp ground paprika
- 1/4 tsp ground cloves
- 1/4 tsp ground nutmeg
- 1/4 tsp cayenne pepper (non-compulsory, for heat)
- Salt and pepper to taste
- 1 can (14 oz) diced tomatoes
- 1 cup of low-sodium chicken broth
- 1/4 cup of dried apricots, chop-up
- 1/4 cup of green olives, pitted
- 2 tbsp chop-up fresh cilantro, for garnish
- Cooked couscous

Instructions:

1. In a big skillet or tagine, warm up the olive oil over medium heat. Add chop-up garlic and chop-up onion. Simmer for about 5 minutes, or until tender.
2. When the chicken pieces are added to the skillet, season them with salt, pepper, cayenne pepper (if using), ground cumin, ground coriander, ground cinnamon, ground ginger, ground turmeric, ground paprika, ground cloves, and ground nutmeg. Cook until all sides of the chicken are browned.
3. Add chop-up dried apricots, green olives, chicken stock, and diced tomatoes. Heat through to a simmer.
4. Turn the heat down to low, cover, and simmer until the chicken is cooked and the flavors are blended, about 1 hr, stirring now and again.
5. Serve hot with chop-up fresh cilantro as a garnish over cooked rice.

Nutrition Info (per serving):

Calories: 320 Protein: 28g Carbohydrates: 22g Fat: 14g Fiber: 4g

Prep Time: 20 min

Cook Time: 30 min

Servings: 4

Points Values: 4 per serving

Ingredients:

- 4 bell peppers (any color), halved and seeds removed
- 1 cup of cooked quinoa
- 1 can (15 oz) black beans, drained and rinsed
- 1 cup of corn kernels
- 1 cup of diced tomatoes
- 1/2 cup of diced onion
- 1/2 cup of diced bell pepper
- 2 cloves garlic, minced
- 1 tsp ground cumin
- 1 tsp chili powder
- Salt and pepper to taste
- 1/2 cup of shredded cheddar cheese (non-compulsory)
- Chop-up fresh cilantro for garnish (non-compulsory)
- Salsa

Instructions:

1. Turn the oven on to 375°F. Lightly grease a baking dish big enough to accommodate the bell pepper halves.
2. Cooked rice or quinoa, black beans, corn kernels, diced tomatoes, diced onion, diced bell pepper, chop-up garlic, ground cumin, chili powder, salt, and pepper should all be mixed in a big dish.
3. Gently press down to stuff the quinoa and veggie mixture into every half of the bell pepper.
4. Fill the baking dish with the stuffed bell peppers. Top the stuffed peppers with shredded cheddar cheese, if you'd like.
5. Bake the baking dish for 25 min in a preheated oven covered with aluminum foil.
6. After 5 more min, or until the peppers are soft and the mixture is thoroughly heated, remove the cover and continue baking.
7. Serve hot with chop-up fresh cilantro as a garnish and, if preferred, salsa or hot sauce on the side.

Nutrition Info (per serving):

Calories: 280

Protein: 12g Carbohydrates: 50g Fat: 4g Fiber: 10g

Prep Time: 20 min

Cook Time: 10 min

Servings: 4

Points Values: 6 per serving

Ingredients:

- 1 lb white fish fillets
- 2 tbsp olive oil
- 1 tsp ground cumin
- 1 tsp chili powder
- 1/2 tsp smoked paprika
- Salt and pepper to taste
- 8 small corn tortillas
- 1 avocado, mashed
- 1/4 cup of Greek yogurt
- 1 tbsp lime juice
- 1/4 cup of chop-up fresh cilantro
- Shredded cabbage
- Split radishes
- Split jalapeños
- Lime wedges for serving

Instructions:

1. Grill at a medium-high temperature.
2. To make a spice rub, mix olive oil, chili powder, smoked paprika, ground cumin, salt, and pepper in a small bowl.
3. Coat the fish fillets with the spice mixture.
4. The fish fillets should be cooked through and flaky after 3–4 min on every side of the grill.
5. On the grill, reheat the corn tortillas for approximately 30 seconds on every side.
6. To prepare avocado cream, mix Greek yogurt, mashed avocado, chopped-up cilantro, and lime juice in a separate bowl.
7. Layer grilled fish, split radishes, split jalapeños, shredded cabbage or lettuce, and avocado cream on top of the warm tortillas to assemble the tacos.
8. Lime wedges should be served alongside.

Nutrition Info (per serving):

Calories: 320

Protein: 25g Carbohydrates: 25g Fat: 14g Fiber: 6g

Prep Time: 30 min

Cook Time: 30 min

Servings: 6

Points Values: 8 per serving

Ingredients:

- 1 lb jumbo pasta shells
- 1 lb ground chicken
- 2 cups of ricotta cheese
- 1 cup of finely grated Parmesan cheese
- 1 cup of shredded mozzarella cheese
- 1 egg
- 2 cups of chop-up spinach
- 2 cloves garlic, minced
- 1 tsp dried basil
- 1 tsp dried oregano
- Salt and pepper to taste
- 2 cups of marinara sauce

Instructions:

1. Turn the oven on to 375°F. In a baking dish that measures 9 by 13 inches, spread the butter.
2. According to the package directions, cook the enormous pasta shells. After draining, set away.
3. Cook the ground chicken in a pan over medium heat until it stops being pink. Eliminate extra fat.
4. Cooked ground chicken, ricotta cheese, finely grated Parmesan cheese, shredded mozzarella cheese, egg, chop-up spinach, chop-up garlic, dried basil, dried oregano, salt, and pepper should all be mixed in a large mixing dish.
5. Place the cooked pasta shells in the baking dish that has been preheated, then stuff everyone with the chicken and cheese mixture.
6. Drizzle the filled shells with marinara sauce.
7. Bake the baking dish for 25 min in a preheated oven covered with aluminum foil.
8. After five more min, or until the cheese is melted and bubbling, remove the foil and continue baking.
9. Warm up the food.

Nutrition Info (per serving):

Calories: 450

Protein: 30g Carbohydrates: 35g Fat: 20g Fiber: 3g

Prep Time: 15 min

Cook Time: 25 min

Servings: 4

Points Values: 5 per serving

Ingredients:

- 1 tbsp olive oil
- 1 onion, diced
- 2 cloves garlic, minced
- 1 tbsp finely grated ginger
- 2 tbsp Thai red curry paste
- 4 cups of chicken
- 1 can (14 oz) coconut milk
- 2 tbsp soy sauce
- 1 tbsp brown sugar
- 1 red bell pepper, thinly split
- 1 yellow bell pepper, thinly split
- 1 cup of split mushrooms
- 1 cup of split carrots
- 1 cup of broccoli florets
- 1 cup of cooked chicken, shredded (non-compulsory)
- Juice of 1 lime
- Chop-up fresh cilantro for garnish
- Cooked rice

Instructions:

1. Warm up the olive oil in a big pot over medium heat. Add diced onion and simmer for about 5 min, or until softened.
2. Stir in the finely grated ginger, chop-up garlic, and Thai red curry paste. Cook until aromatic, one to two min.
3. Add the soy sauce, brown sugar, coconut milk, and chicken. Simmer after stirring to blend flavors.
4. Toss in the broccoli florets, split carrots, split bell peppers, and split mushrooms. Simmer the vegetables for 15 to 20 min, or until they are soft.
5. Add cooked chicken that has been shredded to the soup, if using, and stir until heated through.
6. Take off the heat and mix in the lime juice.
7. Serve hot with chop-up fresh cilantro on top of cooked rice.

Nutrition Info (per serving):

Calories: 320 Protein: 12g Carbohydrates: 20g Fat: 22g Fiber: 4g

Prep Time: 10 min

Cook Time: 40 min

Servings: 4

Points Values: 6 per serving

Ingredients:

- 1 tbsp olive oil
- 1 onion, diced
- 2 cloves garlic, minced
- 8 oz mushrooms, split
- 1 cup of pearl barley
- 1/2 cup of dry white wine (non-compulsory)
- 4 cups of vegetable broth
- 1/4 cup of finely grated Parmesan cheese
- 2 tbsp chop-up fresh parsley
- Salt and pepper to taste

Instructions:

1. In a big skillet or pot, warm up the olive oil over medium heat. Add diced onion and simmer for about 5 min, or until softened.
2. Split mushrooms and chopped-up garlic should be added to the skillet. Simmer the mushrooms for 7 to 8 min, or until they are soft and golden brown.
3. Cook the pearl barley for two to three min, or until it begins to faintly toast.
4. Add the dry white wine, if using, and heat until the liquid is absorbed.
5. Add the vegetable broth gradually, half a cup at a time, stirring constantly and letting the liquid absorb completely before adding more. Cook for 30 to 35 min, or until barley is creamy and soft.
6. Add the chop-up fresh parsley and the finely grated Parmesan cheese. Toss in some salt and pepper and season to taste.
7. If preferred, top with more Parmesan cheese and parsley and serve hot.

Nutrition Info (per serving):

Calories: 280

Protein: 8g Carbohydrates: 45g Fat: 6g Fiber: 8g

SPINACH AND FETA STUFFED PORTOBELLO MUSHROOMS

Prep Time: 15 min

Cook Time: 20 min

Servings: 4

Points Values: 4 per serving

Ingredients:

- 4 large Portobello mushrooms
- 2 cups of chopped, fresh spinach
- 1/2 cup of crumbled feta cheese
- 2 cloves garlic, minced
- 2 tbsp olive oil
- Salt and pepper to taste

Instructions:

1. Set oven temperature to 375°F. Line a baking sheet with parchment paper.
2. With a spoon, carefully remove the stems from the Portobello mushrooms and remove the gills.
3. In a skillet set over medium heat, warm the olive oil. Add the chop-up spinach and chop garlic. Cook for two to three min, or until the spinach has wilted.
4. Take the skillet off of the burner and add the feta cheese crumbles.
5. To fill the caps of the Portobello mushrooms, equally distribute the spinach and feta mixture among them.
6. Stuffed mushrooms should be put on the ready baking sheet. Add pepper and salt for seasoning.
7. Bake for 15 to 20 min, or until cheese is melted and mushrooms are soft, in a preheated oven.
8. Warm up the food.

Nutrition Info (per serving):

Calories: 120

Protein: 5g Carbohydrates: 6g Fat: 9g Fiber: 2g

Prep Time: 15 min

Cook Time: 25 min

Servings: 4

Points Values: 6 per serving

Ingredients:

- 1 cup of quinoa, rinsed
- 2 cups of mixed vegetables chop-up
- 2 tbsp olive oil
- Salt and pepper to taste
- 2 tbsp balsamic vinegar
- 1 tbsp honey
- 1/4 cup of chop-up fresh basil
- 1/4 cup of crumbled feta cheese (non-compulsory)

Instructions:

1. Set oven temperature to 400°F. Line a baking sheet with parchment paper.
2. Mix chop-up veggies, olive oil, salt, and pepper in a bowl. Line the baking sheet with them and spread them out.
3. Bake the vegetables for 20 to 25 min in a preheated oven, or until they are soft and have a hint of caramelization.
4. Cook quinoa in a pot as directed on the package.
5. To make the dressing, mix honey and balsamic vinegar in a small basin.
6. Cooked quinoa, dressing, chop-up fresh basil, and roasted veggies should all be mixed in a big dish. Toss until thoroughly mixed.
7. Before serving, top the salad with crumbled feta cheese, if preferred.
8. Warm up and serve.

Nutrition Info (per serving):

Calories: 280

Protein: 6g

Carbohydrates: 36g

Fat: 12g Fiber: 5g

Prep Time: 10 min

Cook Time: 25 min

Servings: 4

Points Values: 5 per serving

Ingredients:

- 1 tbsp olive oil
- 1 onion, diced
- 2 cloves garlic, minced
- 1 tbsp finely grated ginger
- 1 tbsp curry powder
- 1 tsp ground cumin
- 1 tsp ground coriander
- 1/2 tsp turmeric
- 1/4 tsp cayenne pepper (non-compulsory, for heat)
- One can of chickpeas should be rinsed and drained.
- 1 can (14 oz) diced tomatoes
- 2 cups of fresh spinach leaves
- Salt and pepper to taste
- Cooked rice for serving

Instructions:

1. Heat the olive oil in a big skillet over medium heat. Add diced onion and simmer for about 5 min, or until softened.
2. To the skillet, add the finely grated ginger and chopped-up garlic. Cook until aromatic, one to two min.
3. Add the turmeric, cayenne pepper (if using), ground cumin, ground coriander, and curry powder. Simmer for a further minute.
4. To the skillet, add the diced tomatoes and the drained chickpeas. Mix everything.
5. Simmer for 15 to 20 min over low heat, stirring now and then.
6. Cook the fresh spinach leaves in the skillet for two to three min, or until they have wilted.
7. Toss in some salt and pepper and season to taste.
8. Overcooked rice, served hot.

Nutrition Info (per serving):

Calories: 240 Protein: 9g Carbohydrates: 35g Fat: 8g Fiber: 8g

Prep Time: 15 min

Cook Time: 5 min

Servings: 4

Points Values: 3 per serving

Ingredients:

- 4 medium zucchinis, spiralized into noodles
- 1 cup of cherry tomatoes, halved
- 1/4 cup of basil pesto
- 2 tbsp finely grated Parmesan cheese
- Salt and pepper to taste
- Chop-up fresh basil for garnish

Instructions:

1. A big skillet should be heated to medium heat. Cherry tomatoes and spiralized zucchini noodles should be added to the skillet.
2. Cook, stirring occasionally, until zucchini noodles are barely soft, 3 to 4 min.
3. After removing from the fire, toss the noodles and tomatoes in the basil pesto until well covered.
4. Toss in some salt and pepper and season to taste.
5. Garnish with freshly chopped-up basil and finely grated Parmesan cheese and serve hot.

Nutrition Info (per serving):

Calories: 120

Protein: 5g

Carbohydrates: 10g

Fat: 7g

Fiber: 3g

Prep Time: 30 min
Cook Time: 25 min
Servings: 6
Points Values: 7 per serving

Ingredients:

- 6 large whole wheat tortillas
- 2 medium sweet potatoes, peeled and diced
- 1 can (15 oz) black beans, drained and rinsed
- 1 cup of corn kernels
- 1 red bell pepper, diced
- 1 onion, diced
- 2 cloves garlic, minced
- 1 tsp ground cumin
- 1 tsp chili powder
- 1/2 tsp paprika
- Salt and pepper to taste
- 1 cup of enchilada sauce
- 1 cup of shredded cheese
- Chop-up fresh cilantro for garnish

Instructions:

1. Set oven temperature to 375°F. In a baking dish that measures 9 by 13 inches, spread the butter.
2. In a skillet set over medium heat, warm the olive oil. Cook the sweet potatoes in diced form for 8 to 10 min, or until they are tender.
3. To the skillet, add the diced onion, chopped garlic, diced red bell pepper, ground cumin, paprika, chili powder, salt, and pepper. Simmer the veggies for 5 min or until they are soft.
4. Add corn kernels and black beans and stir. Simmer for a further two to three min.
5. To make the whole wheat tortillas malleable, reheat them as directed on the package.
6. Place a spoonful of the black bean and sweet potato mixture onto every tortilla. Roll up and put in the baking dish that has been prepared, seam side down.
7. Evenly cover the rolled tortillas with the enchilada sauce.
8. Dredge some cheese shredded on top of the enchiladas.
9. Bake the baking dish for 20 min in a preheated oven covered with aluminum foil.
10. After five more min, or until the cheese is melted and bubbling, remove the foil and continue baking.
11. Before serving, add some freshly cut cilantro as a garnish.

Nutrition Info (per serving):

Calories: 320 Protein: 12g Carbohydrates: 45g Fat: 10g Fiber: 8g

Prep Time: 20 min

Cook Time: 30 min

Servings: 4

Points Values: 5 per serving

Ingredients:

- Peel and chop in half four large bell peppers
- 1 cup of cooked quinoa
- One can of chickpeas should be rinsed and drained.
- 1 cup of diced tomatoes
- 1/2 cup of chop-up Kalamata olives
- 1/4 cup of crumbled feta cheese
- 2 tbsp chop-up fresh parsley
- 2 tbsp olive oil
- 1 tbsp lemon juice
- 2 cloves garlic, minced
- Salt and pepper to taste

Instructions:

1. Set oven temperature to 375°F. Lightly grease a baking dish big enough to accommodate the bell pepper halves.
2. Mix cooked quinoa, chickpeas, diced tomatoes, chop-up feta cheese, chop-up fresh parsley, chop-up Kalamata olives, lemon juice, olive oil, salt, and pepper in a big bowl.
3. Gently press the quinoa and Mediterranean mixture into the hollowed-out bell pepper halves.
4. Fill the baking dish with the stuffed bell peppers.
5. Bake the baking dish for 20 min in a preheated oven covered with aluminum foil.
6. After removing the foil, roast the peppers for a further 10 min, or until they are soft.
7. Warm up the food.

Nutrition Info (per serving):

Calories: 280

Protein: 10g Carbohydrates: 35g Fat: 12g Fiber: 9g

Prep Time: 15 min

Cook Time: 10 min

Servings: 4

Points Values: 3 per serving

Ingredients:

- 1 head cauliflower, riced
- 2 tbsp sesame oil
- 2 cloves garlic, minced
- 1 cup of mixed vegetables
- 2 eggs, beaten
- 2 tbsp low-sodium soy sauce
- 2 green onions, chop-up
- Salt and pepper to taste

Instructions:

1. Sesame oil should be heated over medium heat in a big skillet. Add the chopped garlic and simmer for one minute, or until fragrant.
2. Stir-fry the mixed vegetables in the skillet for three to four min, or until they are soft.
3. After pushing the veggies to one side of the skillet, fill the vacant area with the beaten eggs. Cook the eggs through by scrambling them.
4. Add soy sauce and riced cauliflower and stir. Cook, stirring regularly, for a further 3–4 minutes, or until the cauliflower is soft.
5. After taking off the heat, add the chop-up green onions. Toss in some salt and pepper and season to taste.
6. Serve as a main course, hot.

Nutrition Info (per serving):

Calories: 150

Protein: 6g

Carbohydrates: 10g

Fat: 9g Fiber: 4g

Prep Time: 20 min

Cook Time: 40 min

Servings: 4

Points Values: 4 per serving

Ingredients:

- 1 large eggplant, split into rounds
- 2 tomatoes, split
- 1 onion, thinly split
- 2 cloves garlic, minced
- 2 tbsp olive oil
- 1 tsp dried oregano
- 1 tsp dried basil
- Salt and pepper to taste
- 1/4 cup of finely grated Parmesan cheese (non-compulsory)
- Chop-up fresh parsley for garnish

Instructions:

1. Set oven temperature to 375°F. Spread some olive oil on a baking dish.
2. Place the eggplant slices in the baking dish's bottom in a single layer.
3. Add thinly split onion and tomatoes to the top of the eggplant slices.
4. Add some chopped garlic to the veggies. Pour some olive oil over it.
5. Add salt, pepper, dried oregano, and dried basil for seasoning.
6. Finely grated Parmesan cheese can be added if desired.
7. Bake the vegetables for 35 to 40 min in a preheated oven, or until they are soft and have a light brown color.
8. Take out of the oven and sprinkle some freshly chopped-up parsley on top before serving.

Nutrition Info (per serving):

Calories: 120

Protein: 3g

Carbohydrates: 12g

Fat: 7g Fiber: 5g

Prep Time: 15 min

Cook Time: 45 min

Servings: 6

Points Values: 4 per serving

Ingredients:

- 1 cup of dried lentils, rinsed
- 4 cups of vegetable broth
- 1 onion, diced
- 2 carrots, diced
- 2 stalks celery, diced
- 2 cloves garlic, minced
- 1 can (14 oz) diced tomatoes
- 1 tsp dried thyme
- 1 tsp dried rosemary
- Salt and pepper to taste
- Chop-up fresh parsley for garnish

Instructions:

1. Put the vegetable broth and dried lentils in a big pot. Bring over high heat to a boil.
2. Once the lentils are soft, reduce the heat to low, cover, and simmer for 20 to 25 min.
3. Heat the olive oil in a different pot over medium heat. Add the chopped garlic, diced onion, carrots, and celery. Simmer the vegetables for 5 to 7 min, or until they are tender.
4. Add chop-up tomatoes, salt, pepper, dry thyme, and dried rosemary and stir. Simmer for five more min.
5. When the vegetables are in the pot, add the cooked lentils and vegetable broth. Mix everything.
6. For another 15 to 20 min, simmer while covered to let the flavors mix.
7. Garnish with freshly cut parsley and serve hot.

Nutrition Info (per serving):

Calories: 180

Protein: 10g Carbohydrates: 30g Fat: 2g Fiber: 8g

Prep Time: 15 min

Cook Time: 10 min

Servings: 6

Points Values: 5 per serving

Ingredients:

- 1 cup of orzo pasta
- 1 cucumber, diced
- 1 bell pepper, diced
- 1/2 red onion, thinly split
- 1/2 cup kalamata olives, pitted and halved
- 1/2 cup of crumbled feta cheese
- 1/4 cup of chop-up fresh parsley
- 2 tbsp olive oil
- 2 tbsp lemon juice
- 1 tsp dried oregano
- Salt and pepper to taste

Instructions:

1. Follow the directions on the package to cook the orzo pasta. After draining, rinse under cold water.
2. Cooked orzo pasta, diced bell pepper, diced cucumber, thinly split red onion, half-oz Kalamata olives, crumbled feta cheese, and chopped-up fresh parsley should all be mixed in a big bowl.
3. To make the dressing, mix the olive oil, lemon juice, dried oregano, salt, and pepper in a small bowl.
4. After adding the dressing to the salad, stir to fully incorporate.
5. Present cold.

Nutrition Info (per serving):

Calories: 220

Protein: 6g

Carbohydrates: 30g

Fat: 9g Fiber: 3g

LEMON GARLIC BUTTER SHRIMP SKEWERS

Prep Time: 15 min

Cook Time: 10 min

Servings: 4

Points Values: 3 per serving

Ingredients:

- One pound of large shrimp, deveined and shell-free
- 2 tbsp olive oil
- 3 cloves garlic, minced
- Zest of 1 lemon
- Juice of 1 lemon
- 2 tbsp chop-up fresh parsley
- Salt and pepper to taste
- Lemon wedges for serving

Instructions:

1. Grill at a medium-high temperature.
2. Olive oil, chopped garlic, lemon zest, lemon juice, chopped parsley, salt, and pepper should all be mixed in a bowl.
3. Assemble shrimp using skewers.
4. Apply the combination of lemon garlic butter to the shrimp skewers.
5. Shrimp skewers should be cooked for two to three min on every side, or until they are opaque and pink.
6. Take off of the grill and serve hot with wedges of lemon.

Nutrition Info (per serving):

Calories: 180

Protein: 22g

Carbohydrates: 2g Fat: 9g Fiber: 0g

Prep Time: 10 min

Cook Time: 15 min

Servings: 4

Points Values: 4 per serving

Ingredients:

- 4 cod fillets
- 2 tbsp olive oil
- 2 cloves garlic, minced
- 1/4 cup of breadcrumbs
- 2 tbsp chop-up fresh parsley
- 1 tbsp chop-up fresh thyme
- 1 tbsp chop-up fresh rosemary
- Zest of 1 lemon
- Salt and pepper to taste
- Lemon wedges for serving

Instructions:

1. Turn the oven on to 400°F. Coat a baking dish in oil.
2. Cod fillets should be placed in the prepared baking dish.
3. To make the crust, mix the olive oil, breadcrumbs, chop-up garlic, chop-up parsley, chop-up thyme, chop-up rosemary, lemon zest, salt, and pepper in a small bowl.
4. Lightly press the crust mixture onto the top of every fish fillet to ensure it adheres evenly.
5. Bake for 12 to 15 min, or until the crust is golden brown and the fish is cooked through, in a preheated oven.
6. Take out of the oven, then serve hot with wedges of lemon.

Nutrition Info (per serving):

Calories: 220

Protein: 26g

Carbohydrates: 5g

Fat: 10g Fiber: 1g

Prep Time: 15 min

Cook Time: 10 min

Servings: 4

Points Values: 5 per serving

Ingredients:

- 4 salmon fillets
- 2 tbsp olive oil
- 1 tsp chili powder
- 1 tsp paprika
- Salt and pepper to taste
- 1 mango, peeled and diced
- 1/2 red onion, diced
- 1 jalapeño, seeded and minced
- Juice of 1 lime
- 2 tbsp chop-up fresh cilantro

Instructions:

1. Grill at a medium-high temperature.
2. Mix the olive oil, paprika, chili powder, salt, and pepper in a small bowl.
3. Apply the olive oil mixture to the salmon fillets.
4. Salmon fillets should be cooked on the grill for 4–5 min on every side, or until a fork can easily pierce them.
5. Mango salsa is made by combining chop-up cilantro, lime juice, chop-upjalapeño, diced mango, and diced red onion in a separate bowl.
6. Top cooked salmon with mango salsa and serve hot.

Nutrition Info (per serving):

Calories: 280

Protein: 24g

Carbohydrates: 10g

Fat: 16g

Fiber: 2g

Prep Time: 15 min

Cook Time: 0 min

Servings: 4

Points Values: 2 per serving

Ingredients:

- 2 cans (5 oz every) tuna, drained
- 1/4 cup of mayonnaise
- 2 tbsp Sriracha sauce (adjust to taste)
- 1 tbsp soy sauce
- 1 tsp sesame oil
- 1 tsp rice vinegar
- 1/4 cup of chop-up green onions
- 1/4 cup of chop-up fresh cilantro
- 1/4 cup of shredded carrots
- 8 large lettuce leaves

Instructions:

1. The drained tuna, mayonnaise, Sriracha sauce, soy sauce, sesame oil, and rice vinegar should all be thoroughly mixed in a bowl.
2. Add the chop-up cilantro, green onions, and shredded carrots and stir.
3. Spoon a combination of tuna onto leaves of lettuce.
4. To make lettuce wraps, roll up the leaves.

Nutrition Info (per serving):

Calories: 180

Protein: 17g

Carbohydrates: 4g

Fat: 11g

Fiber: 1g

Prep Time: 15 min

Cook Time: 20 min

Servings: 4

Points Values: 4 per serving

Ingredients:

- 4 halibut fillets
- 2 tbsp olive oil
- 2 cloves garlic, minced
- 1 tsp dried oregano
- 1 tsp dried thyme
- 1 tsp dried rosemary
- 1/2 cup of cherry tomatoes, halved
- 1/4 cup of pitted and halved kalamata olives
- 1/4 cup of crumbled feta cheese
- Salt and pepper to taste
- Lemon wedges for serving

Instructions:

1. Set oven temperature to 375°F. Spread some olive oil on a baking dish.
2. After the baking dish is ready, put the halibut fillets in it.
3. Olive oil, chopped garlic, dried oregano, dried thyme, and dried rosemary should all be mixed in a small bowl.
4. Apply the olive oil mixture to the halibut fillets.
5. Place the halibut fillets in the baking dish with the cherry tomatoes and Kalamata olives arranged around them.
6. Place feta cheese crumbles on top of every halibut fillet.
7. Toss in some salt and pepper and season to taste.
8. Bake the halibut for 15 to 20 min in a preheated oven, or until it is cooked through and flakes readily with a fork.
9. Serve hot with wedges of lemon.

Nutrition Info (per serving):

Calories: 250

Protein: 30g Carbohydrates: 4g Fat: 12g Fiber: 1g

Prep Time: 15 min

Cook Time: 5 min

Servings: 4

Points Values: 3 per serving

Ingredients:

- 1 lb shrimp, peeled and deveined
- 1 tbsp olive oil
- Salt and pepper to taste
- 4 cups of mixed salad greens
- 1 avocado, diced
- 1 cup of cherry tomatoes, halved
- 1/4 cup of split red onion
- 2 tbsp chop-up fresh cilantro
- Juice of 1 lime

Instructions:

1. The olive oil should be warmed in a skillet set over medium heat. Add some salt and pepper to the shrimp.
2. When the shrimp are opaque and pink, add them to the skillet and cook for two to three min on every side.
3. Mix the chop-up fresh cilantro, diced avocado, halved cherry tomatoes, split red onion, and mixed salad greens in a big bowl.
4. Toss in some cooked shrimp with salad.
5. Add the lime juice to the salad and gently toss to mix.
6. Serve right away.

Nutrition Info (per serving):

Calories: 220

Protein: 20g

Carbohydrates: 10g

Fat: 12g

Fiber: 5g

Prep Time: 10 min

Cook Time: 15 min

Servings: 4

Points Values: 5 per serving

Ingredients:

- 4 salmon fillets
- 1/4 cup of low-sodium soy sauce
- 2 tbsp honey
- 1 tbsp rice vinegar
- 1 clove garlic, minced
- 1 tsp finely grated ginger
- Sesame seeds for garnish
- Split green onions for garnish

Instructions:

1. Turn the oven on to 400°F. Line a baking sheet with parchment paper.
2. Low-sodium soy sauce, honey, rice vinegar, finely grated ginger, and chopped garlic should all be mixed in a small saucepan. Simmer for two to three min, or until slightly thickened, over medium heat.
3. Put the salmon fillets onto the baking sheet that has been prepared.
4. Saving some of the teriyaki sauce for later, brush the salmon fillets with it.
5. Bake the salmon for 12 to 15 min in a preheated oven, or until it is cooked through and flakes easily with a fork.
6. Use the leftover teriyaki sauce to coat the grilled fish.
7. Before serving, garnish with split green onions and sesame seeds.

Nutrition Info (per serving):

Calories: 300

Protein: 24g

Carbohydrates: 10g

Fat: 15g

Fiber: 1g

Prep Time: 10 min

Cook Time: 10 min

Servings: 4

Points Values: 4 per serving

Ingredients:

- 4 trout fillets
- 2 tbsp olive oil
- Zest of 1 lemon
- Juice of 1 lemon
- 2 cloves garlic, minced
- 1 tbsp chop-up fresh dill
- Salt and pepper to taste
- Lemon wedges for serving

Instructions:

1. Grill at a medium-high temperature.
2. Olive oil, lemon zest, lemon juice, chop-up garlic, chop-up fresh dill, salt, and pepper should all be mixed in a small bowl.
3. Use the lemon-dill mixture to coat the fish fillets on both sides.
4. Cook the trout fillets for 4–5 min on every side, or until the fish flake easily when tested with a fork.
5. Take off of the grill and serve hot with wedges of lemon.

Nutrition Info (per serving):

Calories: 220

Protein: 28g

Carbohydrates: 1g

Fat: 12g

Fiber: 0g

Prep Time: 15 min

Cook Time: 10 min

Servings: 4

Points Values: 3 per serving

Ingredients:

- 1 lb scallops
- One pound of asparagus, cut into small pieces after peeling
- 2 tbsp olive oil
- 3 cloves garlic, minced
- 1 tbsp finely grated ginger
- 2 tbsp low-sodium soy sauce
- 1 tbsp oyster sauce
- 1 tsp sesame oil
- 1 tbsp cornstarch
- 1/4 cup of water
- Salt and pepper to taste
- Cooked rice for serving

Instructions:

1. To create the sauce, mix the oyster sauce, sesame oil, low-sodium soy sauce, cornstarch, and water in a small bowl. Put aside.
2. Set the olive oil in a big skillet and heat it over a high heat. Add the finely grated ginger and chopped-up garlic. About one minute of cooking time should do it.
3. Place a single layer of scallops in the skillet. Scallops should cook for two to three min, or until browned on one side.
4. Add the asparagus to the skillet after flipping the scallops. Cook for a further two to three min, or until the asparagus is crisp-tender and the scallops are cooked through.
5. Drizzle the asparagus and scallops with the sauce. To coat, thoroughly stir.
6. Cook until the sauce has thickened, about 1 more min.
7. Toss in some salt and pepper and season to taste.
8. Overcooked rice, served hot.

Nutrition Info (per serving):

Calories: 220 Protein: 25g Carbohydrates: 10g Fat: 8g Fiber: 3g

Prep Time: 10 min

Cook Time: 15 min

Servings: 4

Points Values: 4 per serving

Ingredients:

- 4 tilapia fillets
- 1/4 cup of finely grated Parmesan cheese
- 2 tbsp breadcrumbs
- 2 cloves garlic, minced
- 1 tbsp chop-up fresh parsley
- 1 tbsp olive oil
- Salt and pepper to taste
- Lemon wedges for serving

Instructions:

1. Turn the oven on to 400°F. Lightly coat an oven tray with olive oil.
2. Finely grated Parmesan cheese, breadcrumbs, chop-up garlic, chop-up fresh parsley, olive oil, salt, and pepper should all be mixed in a small basin.
3. Put the tilapia fillets on the baking sheet that has been prepared.
4. To ensure even coating, press the Parmesan mixture onto the top of every tilapia fillet.
5. Bake for 12 to 15 min, or until the crust is golden brown and the tilapia is cooked through, in a preheated oven.
6. Take out of the oven, then serve hot with wedges of lemon.

Nutrition Info (per serving):

Calories: 200

Protein: 25g

Carbohydrates: 3g

Fat: 8g

Fiber: 0g

LEMON ROSEMARY GRILLED CHICKEN

Prep Time: 10 min

Cook Time: 12 min

Servings: 4

Points Values: 4 per serving

Ingredients:

- 4 boneless, skinless chicken breasts
- 2 tbsp olive oil
- Zest of 1 lemon
- Juice of 1 lemon
- 2 cloves garlic, minced
- 1 tbsp chop-up fresh rosemary
- Salt and pepper to taste
- Lemon wedges for serving

Instructions:

1. Olive oil, lemon zest, lemon juice, chop-up garlic, chop-up fresh rosemary, salt, and pepper should all be mixed in a small bowl.
2. Pour the marinade over the chicken breasts in a shallow dish, rotating them to coat all sides equally. Refrigerate the marinated food for a minimum of half an hour.
3. Grill at a medium-high temperature.
4. Take the chicken breasts out of the marinade and throw away any extra marinade.
5. Chicken breasts should be cooked through and no longer pink in the center after grilling them for 6–7 min on every side.
6. Before serving, remove it from the grill and allow it to rest for a few min.
7. Serve hot with wedges of lemon.

Nutrition Info (per serving):

Calories: 220

Protein: 25g Carbohydrates: 2g Fat: 12g Fiber: 0g

Prep Time: 15 min

Cook Time: 35 min

Servings: 4

Points Values: 5 per serving

Ingredients:

- Remove the seeds and cut four large bell peppers in half lengthwise.
- 1 lb ground turkey
- 1 onion, chop-up
- 2 cloves garlic, minced
- 2 cups of baby spinach
- 1 cup of cooked quinoa
- 1 tsp dried oregano
- 1 tsp dried basil
- Salt and pepper to taste
- 1 cup of shredded mozzarella cheese

Instructions:

1. Turn the oven on to 375°F. Spread some olive oil on a baking dish.
2. After the baking dish is ready, put the bell pepper halves in it.
3. Ground turkey, chop-up onion, and chopped garlic should all be cooked in a skillet over medium heat until the turkey is no longer pink and the onions are mushy.
4. Add the baby spinach and stir until it wilts.
5. Take the skillet off of the burner and mix in the cooked quinoa, salt, pepper, dried oregano, and dried basil.
6. Divide the mixture of turkey and spinach between every bell pepper half.
7. Every filled pepper should have shredded mozzarella cheese on top of it.
8. Bake the baking dish for 25 min in a preheated oven covered with aluminum foil.
9. After removing the foil, bake for a further ten min, or until the cheese is bubbling and melted.
10. Warm up the food.

Nutrition Info (per serving):

Calories: 350

Protein: 30g Carbohydrates: 20g Fat: 15g Fiber: 5g

Prep Time: 10 min

Cook Time: 25 min

Servings: 4

Points Values: 6 per serving

Ingredients:

- 4 bone-in, skin-on chicken thighs
- Salt and pepper to taste
- 2 tbsp olive oil
- 1/4 cup of balsamic vinegar
- 2 tbsp honey
- 2 cloves garlic, minced
- 1 tsp dried thyme
- 1 tsp dried rosemary

Instructions:

1. Turn the oven on to 400°F.
2. Use salt and pepper to season the chicken thighs.
3. In an ovenproof skillet, warm the olive oil over medium-high heat.
4. Place the skin side down on the chicken thighs and cook for 5 to 6 min, or until the skin is crispy and golden brown.
5. Give the chicken thighs another 2 to 3 min on the other side.
6. Mix the honey, balsamic vinegar, dried thyme, dried rosemary, and chopped-up garlic in a small bowl.
7. Over the chicken thighs in the skillet, drizzle the balsamic glaze.
8. After transferring the skillet to the oven, warm it and bake the chicken thighs for 15 to 20 min, or until they are cooked through and the internal temperature reverses 165°F.
9. Warm up the food.

Nutrition Info (per serving):

Calories: 320

Protein: 20g

Carbohydrates: 10g Fat: 22g Fiber: 0g

Prep Time: 15 min

Cook Time: 15 min

Servings: 4

Points Values: 4 per serving

Ingredients:

- 1 pound of skinless, boneless chicken breasts, diced into small pieces
- 2 tbsp soy sauce
- 1 tbsp cornstarch
- 2 tbsp vegetable oil
- 2 cloves garlic, minced
- 1 tsp finely grated ginger
- 4 cups of broccoli florets
- 1 bell pepper, split
- 1/2 cup of chicken broth
- 2 tbsp oyster sauce
- Cooked rice for serving

Instructions:

1. Mix the cornstarch and soy sauce in a bowl. Coat the chicken pieces by tossing them in.
2. In a big skillet, heat the vegetable oil over high heat.
3. Add the finely grated ginger and chop the garlic to the skillet and heat for one minute or until fragrant.
4. Stir-fry the chicken pieces in the skillet for 5 to 6 min, or until they are browned and cooked through.
5. Add split bell pepper and broccoli florets to the skillet. Sauté the veggies for a further three to four min, or until they are crisp-tender.
6. Mix oyster sauce and chicken broth in a small bowl. Transfer to the skillet and let it cook for one to two min, or until the sauce has slightly thickened.
7. Overcooked rice, served hot.

Nutrition Info (per serving):

Calories: 280

Protein: 25g Carbohydrates: 15g Fat: 12g Fiber: 4g

Prep Time: 15 min

Cook Time: 15 min

Servings: 4

Points Values: 3 per serving

Ingredients:

- 1 pound of skinless, boneless chicken breasts, diced into small pieces
- 1/4 cup of hot sauce
- 2 tbsp unsalted butter, melted
- 1 tbsp olive oil
- 1 tsp garlic powder
- 1/2 tsp paprika
- Salt and pepper to taste
- 8 large lettuce leaves (such as Bibb or iceberg)
- 1/4 cup of blue cheese crumbles (non-compulsory)
- 2 celery stalks, thinly split

Instructions:

1. Mix the spicy sauce, melted butter, olive oil, paprika, garlic powder, salt, and pepper in a small bowl.
2. In a skillet, preheat the heat to medium-high. Add the chicken pieces and heat for 6–7 min, or until browned and cooked through.
3. Cover the cooked chicken in the skillet with the hot sauce mixture. To coat, thoroughly stir.
4. Cook until well cooked, 2 to 3 min more.
5. Spoon a mixture of buffalo chicken onto leaves of lettuce.
6. Add thinly split celery and crumbled blue cheese, if using, on top.
7. Serve right away.

Nutrition Info (per serving, without blue cheese crumbles):

Calories: 220

Protein: 25g

Carbohydrates: 2g

Fat: 12g Fiber: 1g

Prep Time: 10 min

Cook Time: 1 hr 30 min

Servings: 6

Points Values: 2 per serving

Ingredients:

- 1 bone-in, skin-on turkey breast (about 3-4 lbs)
- 2 tbsp olive oil
- 2 cloves garlic, minced
- 1 tbsp chop-up fresh thyme
- 1 tbsp chop-up fresh rosemary
- 1 tbsp chop-up fresh parsley
- Salt and pepper to taste
- 1 lemon, thinly split

Instructions:

1. Turn the oven on to 350°F. Apply some olive oil grease to a roasting pan.
2. Olive oil, chop-up garlic, chop-up fresh thyme, chop-up fresh rosemary, chop-up fresh parsley, salt, and pepper should all be mixed in a small bowl.
3. Fill the roasting pan with the turkey breast.
4. Make sure to coat the turkey breast evenly by rubbing it with the herb mixture.
5. Place slices of lemon on top of the turkey breast.
6. Roast for 1 hr and 30 min in a preheated oven, or until the internal temperature of the thickest portion of the breast, when measured with a meat thermometer, reaches 165°F.
7. Take it out of the oven and allow it to rest for ten to fifteen min before slicing.
8. Warm up the food.

Nutrition Info (per serving):

Calories: 250

Protein: 35g

Carbohydrates: 1g

Fat: 12g Fiber: 0g

Prep Time: 15 min

Cook Time: 20 min

Servings: 4

Points Values: 5 per serving

Ingredients:

- 4 boneless, skinless chicken breasts
- Salt and pepper to taste
- 1/4 cup of all-purpose flour
- 2 tbsp olive oil
- 2 cloves garlic, minced
- 1/2 cup of chicken broth
- 1/4 cup of fresh lemon juice
- 2 tbsp capers, drained
- 2 tbsp unsalted butter
- 2 tbsp chop-up fresh parsley
- Lemon slices for serving

Instructions:

1. Add salt and pepper to chicken breasts for seasoning.
2. Chicken breasts should be floured and the excess shaken off.
3. In a big skillet set over medium-high heat, warm up the olive oil.
4. When the chicken breasts are golden brown and well cooked, add them to the skillet and cook for four to five min on every side. Take out and set aside the chicken from the skillet.
5. Add the chop-garlic to the same skillet and sauté for approximately a minute, or until fragrant.
6. Scrape up any browned bits from the bottom of the skillet as you add the lemon juice and chicken broth.
7. Add capers and cook for an additional two to three min.
8. Once the sauce has slightly thickened and the unsalted butter has melted, turn down the heat to low and stir.
9. After removing the chicken breasts from the skillet, cover them with sauce.
10. Cook the chicken for one minute, or until it is well heated.
11. Overtop, scatter freshly chop-up parsley.
12. Serve hot, garnished with slices of lemon.

Nutrition Info (per serving):

Calories: 320

Protein: 30g Carbohydrates: 5g Fat: 18g Fiber: 1g

Prep Time: 20 min

Cook Time: 10 min

Servings: 4

Points Values: 5 per serving

Ingredients:

- 1 lb boneless, skinless chicken breasts, cut into chunks
- 1 cup of pineapple chunks
- 1/2 cup of BBQ sauce
- 1 tbsp olive oil
- Salt and pepper to taste
- Wooden skewers, soaked in water for 30 min

Instructions:

1. Grill at a medium-high temperature.
2. One way to skewer is to thread bits of chicken and pineapple alternately.
3. Mix olive oil and BBQ sauce in a small bowl. Drizzle the blend onto the skewers.
4. To taste, add salt and pepper to the skewers.
5. Cook the chicken on the skewers for 4–5 min on every side, or until the juices run clear.
6. Warm up the food.

Nutrition Info (per serving):

Calories: 250

Protein: 25g

Carbohydrates: 20g

Fat: 8g

Fiber: 2g

Prep Time: 20 min

Cook Time: 30 min

Servings: 6

Points Values: 6 per serving

Ingredients:

- 1 pound of skinless, boneless chicken breasts, diced into small pieces
- Salt and pepper to taste
- 2 tbsp olive oil
- 8 oz mushrooms, split
- 2 cloves garlic, minced
- 2 tbsp all-purpose flour
- 1 cup of chicken broth
- 1 cup of milk
- 1/2 cup of finely grated Parmesan cheese
- 2 tbsp chop-up fresh parsley
- Cooked pasta for serving (non-compulsory)

Instructions:

1. Turn the oven on to 375°F. Apply a layer of olive oil to a casserole dish.
2. Sprinkle salt and pepper on the chicken pieces.
3. In a big skillet set over medium-high heat, warm up the olive oil. Add the chicken pieces and heat for 6–7 min, or until browned all over. Take out and set aside the chicken from the skillet.
4. Add the chop-up garlic and split mushrooms to the same skillet. Cook for about 5 min, or until mushrooms are soft and golden brown.
5. Dust the garlic and mushrooms with flour. To coat, thoroughly stir.
6. Add the milk and chicken broth gradually while stirring continuously for three to four min, or until the sauce thickens.
7. Once the cheese is melted, stir in the finely grated Parmesan and the chop-up fresh parsley.
8. Add the cooked chicken back to the skillet and mix everything.
9. Spoon the mixture into the ready casserole dish.
10. Bake for 25 to 30 min in a preheated oven, or until the tops are bubbly and golden brown.
11. Serve hot with cooked pasta, if desired.

Nutrition Info (per serving, without pasta):

Calories: 320

Protein: 30g Carbohydrates: 8g Fat: 18g Fiber: 1g

Prep Time: 15 min

Cook Time: 20 min

Servings: 4

Points Values: 4 per serving

Ingredients:

- 1 lb ground turkey
- 1/4 cup of breadcrumbs
- 1 egg
- 2 cloves garlic, minced
- 2 tbsp soy sauce
- 1 tbsp fish sauce
- 1 tbsp brown sugar
- 1 tbsp chop-up fresh basil
- 1 tsp finely grated ginger
- 1/2 tsp crushed red pepper flakes (adjust to taste)
- 2 tbsp vegetable oil
- Cooked rice

Instructions:

1. Turn the oven on to 400°F. Line a baking sheet with parchment paper.
2. Ground turkey, breadcrumbs, egg, chopped garlic, soy sauce, fish sauce, brown sugar, chop-up fresh basil, finely grated ginger, and crushed red pepper flakes should all be thoroughly mixed in a big bowl.
3. Form the ingredients into meatballs with a diameter of roughly one inch.
4. In a big skillet, heat the vegetable oil over medium heat. Cook the meatballs in the skillet for about five min, or until they are browned all over.
5. Move the browned meatballs to the ready baking sheet.
6. Bake for 15 minutes, or until cooked through, in a preheated oven.
7. Overcooked rice, served hot.

Nutrition Info (per serving):

Calories: 280

Protein: 25g Carbohydrates: 10g Fat: 15g Fiber: 1g

CHOCOLATE BANANA MUG CAKE

Prep Time: 5 min

Cook Time: 2 min

Servings: 1

Points Values: 7

Ingredients:

- 1 ripe banana, mashed
- 2 tbsp cocoa powder
- 2 tbsp flour
- 1 tbsp sugar
- 1/4 tsp baking powder
- Pinch of salt
- 2 tbsp milk
- 1 tbsp vegetable oil
- 1/4 tsp vanilla extract
- Non-compulsory toppings: split banana, chocolate chips, whipped cream

Instructions:

1. Mash the banana and add the flour, sugar, baking powder, cocoa powder, and salt to a microwave-safe mug. Blend thoroughly.
2. Fill the mug with milk, vegetable oil, and vanilla extract. Get the batter smooth by mixing it.
3. Cook the cake for one to two min on high, or until it is well cooked.
4. Before consuming, allow it to cool for a short while.
5. Add chocolate chips and split bananas on top, if you'd like.

Nutrition Info (per serving):

Calories: 380

Protein: 5g

Carbohydrates: 55g

Fat: 17g Fiber: 7g

Prep Time: 10 min

Cook Time: 0 min

Servings: 2

Points Values: 4 per serving

Ingredients:

- 1 cup of Greek yogurt
- Zest of 1 lemon
- 1 tbsp honey
- 1 cup of mixed berries
- 1/4 cup of granola

Instructions:

1. Gently stir together Greek yogurt, honey, and lemon zest in a small bowl until thoroughly blended.
2. Arrange the Greek yogurt mixture, mixed berries, and granola in serving glasses or jars.
3. Layers are repeated until the glasses are full.
4. Serve right away and put in the fridge until you're ready to eat.

Nutrition Info (per serving):

Calories: 200

Protein: 10g

Carbohydrates: 30g

Fat: 5g

Fiber: 3g

Prep Time: 15 min

Cook Time: 25 min

Servings: 12

Points Values: 3 per serving

Ingredients:

- 8 oz reduced-fat cream cheese, softened
- 1/4 cup of sugar
- 1 egg
- 1 tsp vanilla extract
- 12 reduced-fat vanilla wafer cookies
- Fresh berries for garnish (non-compulsory)

Instructions:

1. Turn the oven on to 350°F. Line a muffin pan with paper liners.
2. Beat the softened cream cheese, sugar, egg, and vanilla extract together until smooth in a mixing dish.
3. In every muffin cup, place a vanilla wafer cookie in the bottom.
4. Evenly spoon the cream cheese mixture over the cookies in a muffin pan.
5. Bake for 20 to 25 min, or until the cheesecake is firm and has a hint of color on top, in a preheated oven.
6. Take out of the oven and allow to cool down fully.
7. If preferred, garnish with fresh berries before serving.

Nutrition Info (per serving):

Calories: 120

Protein: 3g

Carbohydrates: 12g

Fat: 6g

Fiber: 0g

Prep Time: 15 min

Cook Time: 35 min

Servings: 6

Points Values: 6 per serving

Ingredients:

- 4 cups of diced apples
- 1 tbsp lemon juice
- 1/4 cup of sugar
- 1/2 tsp ground cinnamon
- 1/4 tsp ground nutmeg
- 1/4 cup of all-purpose flour
- 1/4 cup of rolled oats
- 2 tbsp brown sugar
- 2 tbsp unsalted butter, melted

Instructions:

1. Turn the oven on to 375°F. Use cooking spray or butter to grease a baking dish.
2. Diced apples should be nicely covered after being tossed in a big basin with sugar, nutmeg, cinnamon, and lemon juice. Place in the baking dish that has been prepared.
3. Melted butter, brown sugar, rolled oats, and flour should all be mixed in a single bowl. Stir until crumbly.
4. Entirely cover the apples in the baking dish with the crumb mixture.
5. Bake for 30 to 35 min in a preheated oven, or until the apples are soft and the topping is golden brown.
6. Before serving, remove from the oven and allow it to cool slightly.
7. Warm up and serve with a scoop of vanilla ice cream, if desired.

Nutrition Info (per serving):

Calories: 180

Protein: 2g

Carbohydrates: 30g

Fat: 7g Fiber: 3g

Prep Time: 15 min

Cook Time: 15 min

Servings: 12 mini pies

Points Values: 4 per serving

Ingredients:

- One and a half cups of crushed graham crackers
- 1/4 cup of sugar
- 6 tbsp unsalted butter, melted
- 3/4 cup of fresh lime juice
- Zest of 2 limes
- 2 large eggs
- 1 can (14 oz) sweetened condensed milk
- Whipped cream and lime slices for garnish (non-compulsory)

Instructions:

1. Turn the oven on to 350°F. Paper liners should be used to line a 12-cup of muffin pan.
2. Melted butter, sugar, and graham cracker crumbs should all be mixed in a mixing basin. Blend until thoroughly blended.
3. Every muffin cup should have the graham cracker mixture firmly pressed into the bottom and up the sides.
4. Mix lime juice, zest, eggs, and sweetened condensed milk in a separate mixing dish and whisk until well mixed.
5. Evenly distribute the lime mixture among the muffin liners.
6. Bake for 12 to 15 min, or until set, in a preheated oven.
7. Take out of the oven and allow to cool down fully.
8. Before serving, place in the refrigerator for at least one hour.
9. If preferred, garnish with lime slices and whipped cream before serving.

Nutrition Info (per serving):

Calories: 250

Protein: 4g

Carbohydrates: 34g Fat: 11g Fiber: 0g

Prep Time: 15 min

Cook Time: 25 min

Servings: 16 brownies

Points Values: 5 per serving

Ingredients:

- 1/2 cup of unsweetened applesauce
- 1/4 cup of vegetable oil
- 1 cup of sugar
- 2 large eggs
- 1 tsp vanilla extract
- 3/4 cup of all-purpose flour
- 1/2 cup of unsweetened cocoa powder
- 1/2 tsp baking powder
- 1/4 tsp salt

Instructions:

1. Turn the oven on to 350°F. Use cooking spray to grease or line an 8 by 8-inch baking tray with parchment paper.
2. Mix applesauce, vegetable oil, sugar, eggs, and vanilla extract in a mixing dish and whisk until thoroughly blended.
3. Sift flour, baking powder, cocoa powder, and salt in a separate basin.
4. Stirring until just blended, gradually add the dry ingredients to the wet components.
5. Evenly distribute the batter after pouring it into the baking pan.
6. Bake for 20 to 25 min, or until a toothpick inserted in the center comes out clean, in a preheated oven.
7. Take it out of the oven and allow it to cool fully before slicing it into squares.

Nutrition Info (per serving):

Calories: 120

Protein: 2g

Carbohydrates: 20g

Fat: 4g Fiber: 1g

Prep Time: 10 min

Cook Time: 0 min

Servings: 8

Points Values: 2 per serving

Ingredients:

- 2 cups of plain Greek yogurt
- 2 tbsp honey
- 1 tsp vanilla extract
- 1 cup of mixed berries
- 2 tbsp chop-up nuts

Instructions:

1. Line a baking sheet with parchment paper.
2. Mix Greek yogurt, vanilla extract, and honey in a mixing dish and whisk until well-mixed.
3. Evenly spread the Greek yogurt mixture over the baking sheet that has been ready.
4. Gently press chop-up nuts and mixed berries into the yogurt mixture by scattering them on top.
5. Freeze the baking sheet for a minimum of two hrs, or until it becomes hard.
6. Cut the yogurt bark into pieces after it has frozen.
7. Serve as a snack right away.

Nutrition Info (per serving):

Calories: 80

Protein: 5g

Carbohydrates: 10g

Fat: 3g

Fiber: 1g

Prep Time: 15 min

Cook Time: 10 min

Servings: 24 cookies

Points Values: 3 per cookie

Ingredients:

- 1 cup of creamy peanut butter
- 1/2 cup of brown sugar
- 1/4 cup of granulated sugar
- 1 large egg
- 1 tsp vanilla extract
- 1 cup of rolled oats
- 1/2 tsp baking soda
- Pinch of salt

Instructions:

1. Turn the oven on to 350°F. Line a baking sheet with parchment paper.
2. Mix peanut butter, brown sugar, granulated sugar, egg, and vanilla extract in a mixing dish and beat until smooth.
3. Mix baking soda, salt, and rolled oats in a basin.
4. Stirring until thoroughly blended, gradually add the dry ingredients to the peanut butter mixture.
5. Form dough into tbsp-sized balls and arrange them on the baking sheet that has been preheated. Using a fork, flatten every ball into a cross-hatch design.
6. Bake for 8 to 10 min, or until the edges of the cookies are golden brown, in a preheated oven.
7. Take out of the oven and allow to rest for five min on the baking sheet, then move to a wire rack to cool down entirely.

Nutrition Info (per cookie):

Calories: 120

Protein: 3g

Carbohydrates: 10g

Fat: 8g Fiber: 1g

Prep Time: 20 min

Cook Time: 0 min

Servings: 8

Points Values: 6 per serving

Ingredients:

- 1 lb strawberries, hulled and split
- 2 tbsp sugar
- 1 tsp vanilla extract
- 1 cup of heavy cream
- 1/4 cup of powdered sugar
- 1 store-bought angel food cake, cut into cubes

Instructions:

1. Mix sugar, vanilla essence, and split strawberries in a mixing dish. After well stirring, let macerate for ten min.
2. Beat heavy cream and powdered sugar in a separate mixing dish until firm peaks form.
3. Arrange the whipped cream, macerated strawberries, and cubes of angel food cake in a trifle dish or individual serving glasses.
4. Layers should be repeated until all ingredients have been used, then whipped cream should be layered on top.
5. Before serving, place in the refrigerator for at least one hour.

Nutrition Info (per serving):

Calories: 250

Protein: 3g

Carbohydrates: 30g

Fat: 14g

Fiber: 2g]

Prep Time: 15 min

Cook Time: 20 min

Servings: 12 muffins

Points Values: 4 per muffin

Ingredients:

- 2 cups of all-purpose flour
- 1/2 cup of granulated sugar
- 1 tbsp baking powder
- 1/2 tsp salt
- 1 cup of plain Greek yogurt
- 1/4 cup of cooled and melted unsalted butter
- 2 large eggs
- Zest of 1 lemon
- 2 tbsp fresh lemon juice
- 1 tsp vanilla extract
- 1 cup of fresh blueberries

Instructions:

1. Turn the oven on to 375°F. Use cooking spray or paper liners to line a muffin tray.
2. Mix the flour, sugar, baking powder, and salt in a sizable mixing bowl.
3. Blend Greek yogurt, eggs, melted butter, lemon zest, lemon juice, and vanilla essence in a separate dish until smooth.
4. Stirring until just blended, gradually add the wet components to the dry ingredients.
5. Add the fresh blueberries and fold gently.
6. Using a spoon, pour the batter into every muffin tray, filling it to about 3/4 of the way.
7. Bake for 18 to 20 min, or until a toothpick inserted in the center comes out clean, in a preheated oven.
8. Take it out of the oven and allow it to cool in the muffin tray for five min, then take it to a wire rack to cool down fully.

Nutrition Info (per muffin):

Calories: 180 Protein: 5g Carbohydrates: 25g Fat: 6g Fiber: 1g

CONCLUSION

It's important to take stock of our joint journey as we approach the last pages of the Weight Watch New Complete Cookbook 2024. This cookbook is more than just a list of recipes; it's a resource for anybody devoted to using mindful eating to lead a longer, happier life. It's also a mentor, guide, and source of inspiration.

We have examined a wide range of tastes, textures, and cuisines on these pages, all of which have been thoughtfully chosen to adhere to the Weight Watchers philosophy. We've studied nutrition science and learned how eating well-balanced meals can support our physical and mental well-being. Every meal has been created to offer taste without sacrificing flavor, from filling dinners that unite families to full breakfasts that give you energy for the day.

This cookbook is a tribute to the tradition of sustainable, healthful living that the Weight Watchers program has long stood for. It provides nutrient-dense yet quick-and-easy-to-make dishes, acknowledging the changing demands of a modern lifestyle. Since we recognize that everyone has a hectic schedule, our book attempts to make eating healthfully enjoyable and accessible to everybody.

The inclusivity of this cookbook is among its most impressive features. There are recipes that will test your abilities and broaden your culinary repertoire, regardless of your level of experience in the kitchen. You may prepare dishes that are visually attractive and delicious with confidence thanks to the step-by-step directions and helpful tips and tricks.

Additionally, this cookbook highlights how important customization and flexibility are. A key component of the Weight Watchers program is the points system, which lets you modify recipes to fit your unique nutritional requirements and preferences. It empowers you to take charge of your journey towards improved health by encouraging you to make decisions that are in line with your individual health goals.

Finally, it's critical to recognize that the path to wellness is a continuous one. The recipes in these pages are meant to be tools to help you, but the real success is found in the daily choices and habits you create. Never forget to rejoice in your accomplishments, no matter how tiny, and greet every meal with enthusiasm and interest.

The goal of The Weight Watch New Complete Cookbook 2024 is to be a reliable guide for you as you pursue better health. You can use it again and again to discover new favorites and re-visit treasured recipes. Allow it to motivate you to do new things, to enjoy life, and to take care of your family.

We appreciate you letting us share in your culinary adventure. I hope you have many more tasty and healthful meals and that the simple act of sharing food enriches your life. Have fun in the kitchen!